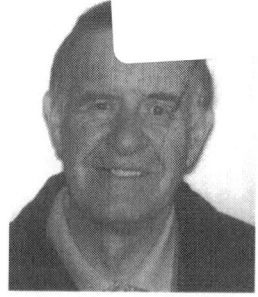

JOHN C MCGREGOR BSc MB ChB FRCS FRCS(Ed) was born in Paisley in 1944. He was educated at Paisley Grammar School and went on to study Medicine at Glasgow University, qualifying with honours in physiology in 1967 and MB ChB with commendation and distinction in Surgery in 1969. He achieved a lifetime ambition and became a Consultant in Plastic Surgery in Edinburgh in 1980, where he remained until retirement from the NHS in 2006. He received training in Plastic Surgery in Canniesburn Hospital, Glasgow, Nottingham City Hospital, and Bangour General Hospital, West Lothian. He also received general surgical training as Hall Fellow in the Western Infirmary, Glasgow, and as a registrar in Stobhill Hospital, also in Glasgow. During this period, he obtained experience in casualty, orthopaedics, and neurosurgery in these hospitals and the Southern General Hospital in Glasgow.

In *My Hidden Self: A Plastic Surgeon's Diary of a Stroke*, John McGregor writes a personal account of his stroke, his experiences at the time and his first year at home. He gives a unique and thought-provoking story of his care from the NHS, the help available and his fight against the odds.

Though he has published over one hundred articles on various topics in medical journals, this is his first in the form of a book. He has appeared on several TV programmes as well as radio discussions, live and recorded. The book is illustrated with photographs and personal paintings that were all done using his non-dominant hand after his stroke.

My Hidden Self

A Plastic Surgeon's Diary of a Stroke

My Hidden Self

A Plastic Surgeon's Diary of a Stroke

John C McGregor

ATHENA PRESS
LONDON

MY HIDDEN SELF
A Plastic Surgeon's Diary of a Stroke
Copyright © John C McGregor 2009

ISBN 978 1 84748 518 2

First published 2009 by
ATHENA PRESS
Queen's House, 2 Holly Road
Twickenham TW1 4EG
United Kingdom

Printed for Athena Press

To my wife, Moira, and children, Trudy and Alan

Acknowledgements

I would like to acknowledge the excellent care and attention I received from Professor Dennis and his staff at ward 55, Western General Hospital, and ward 9, Royal Victoria Hospital, Edinburgh. I am also indebted to the outpatient care at the various clinics in the Western General, including urology, diabetic/hypertension, and gastroenterology. Mr Tolley, Dr Strachan, Dr McNight, and Dr Palmer respectively were the Consultants involved. The care workers and physiotherapists (Dawn, Alison, Kenny, and stroke nurse Sheila), at Astley Ainslie Hospital (Katie and Jane), and McLeod Street Clinic (Julie Hooper) were extremely beneficial as well as being essential to my recovery. Ayla and colleagues were of great help to me in supervising my recovery physiotherapy at the Drumbrae Leisure Club. Emma Sawyer gave further invaluable physiotherapy with home visits. Mr John Lyall and the hospital volunteers helped greatly with computer work and production of pictures from my artwork. Gordon and John, of DMC Computer Services, Barnton, were also of great help. My GP, Dr Patricia Donald was always available to me for advice, liaison, and aftercare – a good example of what a caring and helpful GP should be. Dr David Jolliffe of the Cramond Practice was also involved in my care. Miss Battison provided some excellent dental care.

I would also like to acknowledge the influence of George Bruce's book *Through the Letterbox*, and the dragonfly picture and associated poem, which gave me great motivation to write as well as illustrate this book.

Lastly, I would never have managed so well without the help and encouragement given unselfishly by my wonderful wife, Moira, and my many friends and relatives. My apologies for any omissions.

Contents

About this Book

This account was written by a doctor and a surgeon who suddenly became afflicted by a stroke. It describes events from just before the onset, through his hospital stay and afterwards at home until one year after the stroke. The serious effects resulting are not dismissed, and the author discusses them and how an optimistic approach in his situation was helpful in achieving recovery, as well as the role of others in making this more likely. There is still much ignorance regarding the causes of strokes, the age groups affected, the inpatient procedure, the investigations and treatment, the help available as an outpatient, and the overall life changes that are necessary. This book is designed to help others who are afflicted by strokes and to be of help to those who care for them, and has been written by someone with a unique experience of having worked in the NHS over many years.

Part One
Early Days

The First Hours

Little did I know when I went to bed feeling well on 18 July 2007 that my life was about to change significantly during the following day. At about 4 a.m. I awoke with a strange feeling in my right arm and leg – as if I had been sleeping too long in one position. This was not something I could recall I had ever experienced before. I got out of bed and staggered to the toilet, falling to my right but able to regain balance before returning to bed assisted by my anxious wife, Moira. There were no associated symptoms such as headache, vomiting, chest or abdominal pain – only a vague feeling of unease and sweating. At that time, in spite of my medical background, surprisingly, I did not consider the possibility that I was in process of developing a stroke. Was this self-denial or due to the fact there was no close family history of strokes? I did not smoke or drink alcohol in excess, and I had never been a patient in hospital or off work as a doctor, from resident house officer up to my retirement from the NHS as a consultant plastic surgeon in April 2006 at the age of sixty-two years. Furthermore, from then on, when I continued to work privately as a plastic and cosmetic surgeon during the rest of 2006 and to the time of this event, I had not been required to attend hospital as an inpatient.

This time I really felt distinctly ill at ease and took little per-suasion from Moira that we should call the doctor for advice. Of course, when we telephoned our local practice at that early morning time we were directed to NHS 24! Discussion on the telephone, firstly with a sympathetic-sounding nurse and then a doctor, resulted in the decision that according to my symptoms and signs described calmly and clearly by me, I could wait at home and telephone my own practice at 8.15 a.m. I was not in a position to disagree, but I was left not feeling entirely at ease with the advice given by an unknown doctor who had not, as far as I could ascertain, made a diagnosis. I can see how many people have some worries about NHS 24.

My worries were not over at 8.15 a.m. or later, when two more telephone calls to the local practice at 8.30 and 8.45 produced an engaged tone: very disturbing, especially as I was not getting better, although by this time I had shaved, dressed and could walk unaided though with increasing difficulty. There seemed no point in trying NHS 24 again and though we might have driven to a casualty department where I could have presented as a new patient, it seemed more appropriate to persist with the advice given and contact the local practice. After a tense debate, I persuaded Moira to drive to the practice to find out what the problem of the telephone was; Moira was very reluctant to leave me at home, but given various scenarios this seemed to be the best option. She quickly returned with the information that there had been a power cut at the practice, and this was why there had been a problem with the telephone. The good news was that if I went to the practice immediately I could be seen – and by a GP who knew me.

I managed with some difficulty to get into the car and be driven by Moira the short drive to the practice and then into the GP surgery. She (the doctor) quickly assessed my problem and agreed I should go immediately to be admitted to hospital. To save time, and rather than await an ambulance during the morning rush hour, Moira and I decided to use our car.

I arrived within about twenty-five minutes at the assessment unit in the Western General Hospital at about 10 a.m. though by now I had lost track of time. I was still able to walk with difficulty, and could talk normally, but was now quite concerned about my situation. The area seemed to be full of nurses and patients – some walking, some in chairs, and some in beds. Initially I sat on a chair in a busy corridor but as I was beginning to feel weaker I was put on a bed. I was thirsty but was told by a passing nurse that I 'was not allowed to drink until it had been checked that I could swallow'. This seemed to be unfair, especially since water in jugs was within easy reach, and it seemed an age before someone came to assess me. When this happened it was explained to me that all stroke patients had to do a test swallow in case of difficulties. When this was done, and I had no problems, I was given a welcome drink of cool water.

Various young women, possibly nurses or doctors, then came to see me, examined me, asked questions, and took samples of blood and urine. I was able to respond to questions to demonstrate my name, age, address, date, and medical history. There seemed to me to be no obvious urgency about the way things were being conducted, and for me time seemed to stand still. No doubt things were happening behind the scenes, but for me, and possibly for Moira, it was an anxious time – made worse by the feeling that my right arm and leg were becoming weaker. Word came back that my urine contained sugar and I was diabetic. This was quite a surprise as my GP had tested for this a few weeks before and said I was *not* a diabetic! There was still no word about admission, and this was not explained – a further worry to contend with.

When eventually I was moved, I (and Moira, who presumably had an idea of what was to occur over the next few hours) was admitted to ward 55 – the regional specialist stroke unit in the same hospital. I was kept here for ten days.

In retrospect I can understand why and how things appeared to be progressing irritatingly slowly, as behind the scenes my case was being assessed and discussed carefully and professionally at the highest levels.

Before I was admitted I had major tests and was able to consent for these: a carotid ultrasonic test, an MRI brain scan, and an arterial dye injection study of the vessels supplying my brain. All of these were essential in my view, vital in the understanding and management of a stroke, and need not be feared.

The results of these tests showed that both the carotid arteries in my neck were completely normal. This was the quickest and most comfortable examination, involving application of lubricating oil to my neck and application of a small scanner to the neck. A picture of this Doppler examination was immediately illustrated on a screen.

The next two examinations could in no way be described as either pleasant or comfortable.

Before going into the 'tunnel-like' structure which was the MRI machine, I was told that it might feel claustrophobic but at any time I would be in touch with the outside people by using a hand-held buzzer or by a two-way radio system and could then abort at any time. By this time I seemed to be struggling to climb up on to the trolley which was to be pushed head first into the apparatus, but I managed. When I was completely inside, the door at my feet was closed and I was now enclosed – like an entombment! It was then confirmed with the outside persons that I was comfortable and, if so, the test could begin. I could keep my eyes closed if I wished but should try to keep still. Periodically I was to hear odd clanking sounds which would come between the actual test runs. I chose to keep my eyes closed for most of the time, and initially I did not feel threatened or worried about being enclosed. This comfortable feeling did not continue, as time seemed to last for ever. Several test runs were required, and my bladder needed to be relieved (but could not be without stopping the examination). Also, the tests – each lasting about two minutes – involved me not moving. Perhaps the most disturbing of all was the peculiar metallic clanking, which sounded like some extra-terrestrial beast, and occurred in between each test.

At long last this came to an end and I was freed! The examination had been completed successfully and would – thank goodness – not need to be done again.

I was next wheeled to another area for my final procedure in what seemed a very long and exhausting day. I now had no idea of the time but felt it was mid-afternoon. Though Moira was still around I felt I was not able to talk freely or often enough in order to reassure her; I felt she must be worried. Perhaps she was being kept informed, but I had no way of knowing; besides, in my position there was absolutely nothing I could do about this.

The next stage was conducted in a large area filled with various electrical gadgets and what seemed to be many individuals – nurses, doctors, and technical staff. This was quite daunting, but at the same time reassuring. It was explained that a cannulation of my right femoral artery would be performed in order to inject a radio-opaque dye to visualise my brain arterial system, and possibly do an angioplasty procedure – an unblocking of an artery. I gave my written consent for what was a procedure that could and was quickly undertaken without an anaesthetic. What followed however took much longer, and with the accompaniment of much muffled discussion about 'what to do' etc. None of this I understood, nor was I given an explanation of it at the time. All I learned was that there were 'some problems in visualising all relevant blood vessels', and after what again seemed to be a very long time, it was agreed to stop. By this time, with an intravenous drip in one arm, an indwelling urinary catheter, and a cannula into my right groin and artery, I was more than ready to have a rest in the admission ward. I had no idea of the time – I thought it might be late afternoon – but I no longer cared!

First Thoughts

After a restless night in a strange ward, I awoke early when the day shift nurses appeared and took over from the night staff. This time – about 7 a.m. – was not an hour I was unused to. This, I found out later, was fairly standard in each of the wards I ended up in. The present ward was ward 55, which was situated in the second floor of a relatively modern part of the Western General Hospital in Edinburgh known as the Anne Ferguson Building. Later I found out that this was the main admission ward for strokes in Edinburgh and the Lothians, which reassured me as well as confirming why I had become ill and required admission. The realisation of this was confirmed by the fact that I now found I was unable to move my right leg as well as my right arm and hand. In addition, I was to discover that I was unable to turn or even shift myself up the bed when I slipped down – for this manoeuvre I found I would have to call a nurse to help. More about this later!

Many people who find themselves in my situation, especially having been in good health before, did not smoke or drink alcohol excessively, and whose parents like mine had no history of strokes and both lived to the age of ninety years and did not have strokes, might feel bitter and ask the question, 'Why me?' At no time, either then or subsequently, have I felt this to be an issue as far as I was concerned, but I can readily understand how these could be the thoughts of the average person. For Moira, as well as my relatives and friends, this had been an unexpected and surprising setback, which seemed to be unfair for someone like me.

When I thought about the preceding months I began to consider a few warning signs that might have been significant and, had I paid more attention to them, I might have changed things.

I had decided to retire early from my job as a Consultant Plastic Surgeon in St John's Hospital, West Lothian, in April 2006 after thirty-six years in the NHS, during which time I was never ill or off work. My reasons for retiring were to do with the timing of a suitable pension for senior staff in the NHS, which the Government had just agreed, and the concomitant irritation and frustration caused by the hospital administrators with regard to the massaging of waiting lists and other patient number-oriented statistics. I had felt that the job I had mostly enjoyed had become much less rewarding, and since this was so, and I seemed to be unable to alter this, the time was right for me to go. Since I was able to continue with a modest private practice, including some cosmetic surgery and examination work with the Royal College of Surgeons of Edinburgh and the British Association of Plastic Surgeons, I felt entirely comfortable. The only clinical things that might in retrospect have been of significance were an increasing need to drink water at clinics and between operating cases, concomitant with urgent and more frequent toilet stops! None of this I really thought of as being worrying or needing medical tests or a visit to the GP. Diabetes did not jump out at me!

During March 2007, Moira and I enjoyed a cruise in South America without any health problems, visiting Chile, Peru, and Ecuador. This involved visiting Machu Picchu, at high altitude, and the Galapagos Islands, and involved not inconsiderable physical efforts. At this time the birth of our third grandchild in India was due in April, and a visit to New Delhi was planned in April.

It was during one of my outpatient sessions in private at my room at the local private hospital (Murrayfield Hospital) that I had a sudden episode of double vision and associated dizziness and sweating. This occurred on 25 April. I had no other symptoms such as pain or headache. The nurses and reception staff were so concerned that they called for the 'crash team' to come urgently and examine me. Examination indicated that I had not suffered a heart attack but had a very high blood pressure. I recovered quite quickly but took a taxi home. I was advised to seek an early appointment with my GP, which I arranged. The GP confirmed that my blood pressure was indeed very high and required medication to try and lower it, pointing out that it may take a few months and additional medication. Samples of my blood were taken, and these showed no particular problems: no raised blood sugar, and electrolytes and urea were normal. The level of my serum cholesterol was only slightly raised. It was also confirmed that I could still plan to make the visit to India. As I was a non-smoker and moderate alcohol drinker, no modification to my lifestyle on those accounts was deemed necessary.

The visit to India was one we had done on several occasions and though it involved a long flight and the hot weather, it was not a journey that troubled me. Moira and I had a wonderful time meeting our son, Alan, his beautiful wife Susanna, and of course our new grandson, Joshua! During the stay, I can recall three small short-lived periods of double vision, the last occurring while rushing to departure in the airport.

On return home in June I was reviewed by my GP, who noted that my blood pressure was still too high and suggested I needed more medication and referral to the Blood Pressure Clinic in the Western General Hospital, This was done, and when I attended it was agreed that I required more medication, a 24-hour monitor of my blood pressure, and much to my surprise, management of type 2 diabetes by diet and drugs (but not insulin). The last situation was the result of analysis of a urine and a blood sample taken at the clinic, and required another appointment at the nearby Diabetic Clinic. Attending this confirmed the diabetes and gave me general advice on medication and diet. My eyes were checked by special optic fundus photography, and this showed that there was no evidence of diabetic or hypertensive damage to the blood vessels. None the less, it was quite a shock to discover that I was a diabetic, especially as my GP had told me otherwise! This was based on blood results analysed elsewhere.

During the month of June and early July, I continued to work at my private practice, but for the first time more slowly and much more aware that I had to look after my health. Worrying, I had several minor episodes of dizziness both at home and at the private hospital, but never during operations or clinics. For the first time I considered that an earlier decision to retire from surgery at the end of 2007 or April 2008 might be a reality.

The really worrying episode occurred forty-eight hours before 19 July (the date of my stroke) during a golf match at the Royal

Burgess Golf Club, when at the seventh hole I became aware that I was seeing *two* golf balls! This situation persisted for the next two holes and then cleared completely, such that I was able to complete my round and win the match!

Whether I would have been wiser to not complete my round remains for ever uncertain. It now seems likely that all these strange episodes were what can be called 'transient ischaemic episodes' – a forewarning of a possible stroke.

The First Ten Days in Ward 55, Western General Hospital

My first view of ward 55 showed I was in four-bedded room in a bed on the left-hand side of the entrance to the ward. I was surrounded on each side by bed supports which were designed to keep me from falling or getting out – not that I was capable of moving in order to do this anyway! I was still catheterised so I had no immediate worries regarding this. There was a TV in the room which was situated for general use on a table near the window, which itself had an uninspiring view of the hospital wall. A nurse gave me a small breakfast of toast and a cereal, together with a card to fill in to order meals for the rest of the day and for the next. I was told if this was not done I would not get fed! Fortunately, since I had the full use of my left hand, I could both feed myself and fill in the card by ticks. Most importantly, the nurse showed me a cord with an attached control panel which had a number of controls and which contained a button to press if I needed to call for assistance. This seemed to be extremely reassuring, but subsequent use of this demonstrated that its use was not guaranteed to produce a rapid response; the average time was ten minutes and was probably quicker during the night or when the nurses were not busy in the ward with other patients.

In the ten days I was in this ward I did not get to know my companion patients, partly because some were going home, and partly because I was only kept in the ward 55 for a short time. The first patient, who was in the bed opposite, was a man of about ten years younger than me with a similar type of stroke. He had been in for at least one week before me, and had some problem with his speech. He was slightly more mobile and he was able to get out of bed and onto a wheelchair with a little assistance. The others were older men with varying degrees of disabilities and confusion, but they appeared to be self-mobile. This initial exposure let me know that strokes varied in their severity and could occur in the young as well as the old. (30% of strokes occur in the under-60s.)

Indeed I realised that I had suffered a stroke, but strangely I did not feel annoyed, disappointed or bitter. Further information and confirmation of my situation came early on that first morning, demonstrating both the good and bad of the NHS. The good was illustrated by the Professor in charge of my care, the bad by the actions of two other doctors who came to see me some thirty minutes afterwards in an attempt to change my mind on treatment already agreed with the Professor. I will explain how this arose.

Professor Dennis came in early to see me and introduced himself. This was the first time I can recall seeing him but I was immediately impressed by his approach and directness. He made it quite clear to me from the results of my scans and vascular studies that I had had a series of small infarcts or strokes in the hind part of my brain, and this was associated with a complete blockage of an artery on the left side and partial blockage of another on the right. There was also an unusual vascular abnormality affecting another main artery, which was noted but the significance was uncertain. An attempt to unblock the partially blocked artery by angioplasty had failed and it had not been judged safe to persist with this in case further damage ensued. To help me understand the situation he drew some diagrams, and this was very helpful. He explained that overnight he had been thinking about my case and what should be the best treatment options. He said I could myself determine this to some extent, but thought that further surgery such as insertion of a stent – rather like what is commonly done to increase the flow in coronary arteries – was both experimental and risky in brain vessels. Few such cases had been done, and the results to date were not yet convincing. He would suggest that going with blood thinners and other medications would on balance be a good alternative. Since the femoral line was still in place the option of inserting a stent was still open to me, but he emphasised that it remained my decision.

He gave me a few minutes to think over the facts and I did so very carefully. This of course is no easy thing to do for any patient in my situation. I did not think it was something I could discuss with my wife and family, as this would put great and unfair pressure on all. I was mindful of my own father, who at the age of ninety years had died during an angioplasty procedure for heart disease, and wondered what I would do were it be one of my own family to decide for. I thus opted for the non-operative pathway and told the Professor so. I think he was in agreement! I will forever be grateful to him for his frankness and his clinical judgement.

Imagine how I felt when some thirty minutes later I was faced with two other doctors – possibly radiologists – who came and tried to get me to change my mind and agree to the invasive procedure. With some difficulty I persuaded them that I had decided of my own free will *not* to have further surgical intervention. I felt that this additional pressure was unwarranted as well as deeply unsettling to a patient in my position. I decided to go along with my own gut feelings and trust the wisdom and experience of the Professor. Time would tell if I had made a wise decision and I was prepared to accept this. It could turn out to be the biggest decision of my life.

Having now resolved the above, I now returned to the new circumstances of my admission. I was unable to move much in bed and observed that the only thing I could do with regard to my limbs on the affected side was a tiny muscle flicker on the inner side of my middle finger and a similar one above my knee. Fortunately, I seemed to have no facial or speech difficulties, so communication was not a problem. There did seem to be more sweating down the right of my body – this was to last almost two months more, and proved to be very uncomfortable problem during the night and day. It was I think associated with the site of my stroke in the hindbrain rather than the ward environment, since I did not notice that in others. To help me, a welcome electric fan was obtained for me to use when required. Apart from that I was surprisingly comfortable, was enjoying the ordered meals, and had nice visits from close family (including my son Alan, who had come all the way from India to see me). However, the situation changed with the removal of my catheter and the femoral arterial line a few days after my admission. The latter resulted in a haematoma (blood clot) the size of a small orange in my right groin and upper thigh. This was initially painful but did eventually disappear slowly over the next six months. The removal of the urinary catheter meant I had to try and use a 'bottle' – quite a difficult manoeuvre in bed and with only one hand, especially if there was a degree of urgency on occasion! This situation was to 'dog' me over the next two to three months. It became worse as the nurses decided that since my bowels had not moved after three days, I should be given a laxative! The result was I was given a foul-tasting fluid to drink and an hour or two later – just about when I thought I had escaped – all hell broke loose! First there was a sudden onset of severe abdominal cramps. Secondly, I had to rush to get to the buzzer to call for a nurse, who did not come immediately, and thirdly, with what seemed an eternity I was lifted out of my bed using a sling apparatus, transferred into a wheelchair, moved across the ward to the toilet-cum-shower room, and transferred onto the toilet using the sling method.

On completion there was the reverse process to get me back to bed. Before this there was the embarrassment of the same nurse cleaning me up! This slightly upsetting procedure was to occur at least once more during my stay in ward 55, and was also used when I went to be washed in the shower (usually every second day).

It was not all bad, however, and I was beginning to receive 'get well' cards and messages and wonderful bouquets of flowers from the staff of Murrayfield Hospital and from the British Association of Plastic and Aesthetic Surgeons. I found that I was able to keep myself occupied by observing the work of the ward, trying to unravel the mysteries of sudoku and work with a DVD player which Alan had brought me and used it to view the film *Gladiator,* which Trudy and her husband, Andrew, gave me a loan of.

Of considerable interest and stimulus for me were the visits to the nearby physiotherapy department and assessment by the senior physiotherapist, a lady whose father I knew when I worked in the NHS, and who himself had suffered a stroke. I was initially transported to and from my bed to the physiotherapy room, using the method described for toilet and shower, and to and from the bench I was examined on. The trip was the first out of my room and involved what could be described at that time to be 'an exciting safari', even though it was only a short trip through several doors and corridors! It was confirmed that I could not move my right arm or leg but I had good sensation and more importantly an appreciation of proprioception (awareness of joint and digit position). Of great significance was that I was able to sit up and remain so without the need to be supported. Further visits during this week confirmed that I could be stood up with support but was not able to step forward. I remember her words at this early time and which remained with me during my hospitalisation as a great comfort and stimulus. These were, 'You will definitely walk again, perhaps with a limp,' and, 'Always have a goal to try for by the end of each week.' There is no doubt that for me this gave me a huge psychological lift, even though I was not actually depressed. From that day I had no doubt that someday I would walk again!

Although my visits proved to be few they gave me the first chance to talk freely and comfortably with someone about my stroke and the problems – something that did not seem possible with any of the nursing staff, or even the doctors in the ward, who seemed to be short on the ground as well as familiarity with my case details. None appeared concerned about my colder right foot, or looked at the large slightly painful haematoma in my right groin. (Only once over the next four months was I examined.)

It was in fact the physiotherapist at the end of the week who told me that it would be my last time with her, as I was going to be transferred at the beginning of the next week to the Royal Victoria Hospital, just down the road! This came as quite a shock, as I felt I had established an important helper for my recovery, and no one before, either nurse or doctor, had said I would be moving so soon. She reassured me that the physiotherapy would be continued by others.

Over the next weekend I confirmed with the nurses that it was proposed that I be transferred to ward 9 of the said hospital, and was told this 'was standard for patients who came from my area in Edinburgh'. I was quite resigned to the move and had decided to put my trust in the medical decision, even though I had never been told this by any doctor at this time. Imagine my alarm when my wife and a retired GP visitor both expressed surprise about the proposed transfer during their Saturday night visit, and the latter went so far as to say I should refuse to go! I had decided to go with the move none the less. The GP's view was based wrongly, as it transpired, on the 'reputation' of a separate part of the hospital dating from many years ago.

However, it resulted in some disquiet, and my daughter, Trudy, complained to the medical staff about the lack of information available both to me and the close relatives on the proposed transfer; she received an apology from a junior doctor. Moira, unbeknown to me, made a visit with a friend, Nan Christie, who had herself worked many years ago in the geriatric part of the hospital concerned, and surveyed ward 9 on the Sunday. Their observations were very reassuring, and meant on the night before I was to be transferred all concerned were comfortable about the move. Naturally I still had some anxiety about the unknown!

Part Two

Royal Victoria Hospital, Edinburgh,
until 16 November

First Impressions in a New Abode

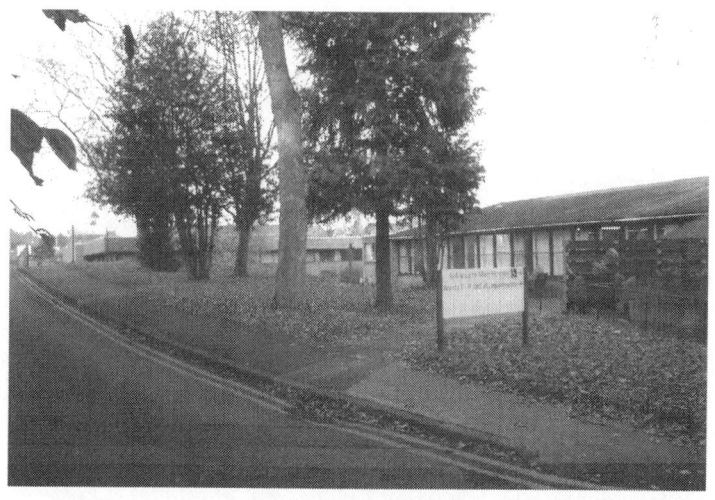

Ward 9, external view. Courtesy of Mr Alf Cattenach

I was transferred by ambulance to my new abode late on the Monday morning and in so doing missed lunch in both hospitals. The journey itself was extremely short as the two hospitals were virtually next to each other. The day was bright and sunny but I still felt apprehensive about the next stage. The ward I was to go to was situated at the far part of a hospital containing wards and patients that included geriatrics and dementia inmates. It was an old hospital situated within a wooded area with walking areas and grassy parts that also contained some enclosed outside gardens – all of which were accessible to patients and visitors.

Ward 9 was named as the 'Stroke Rehabilitation Unit' and was a brightly lit single-storey building at ground level. It had a total of thirty to thirty-two beds and was neatly divided in two by a central area which contained toilets, showers, and nursing rooms and data boards showing patient names and treatment status for each day. The male patients were on the right while the females were on the left, separated by the central area but with access through by a short connection passage. On each side there was a single room, a double room, and two six-bedded areas – blue covers for the 'boys' and pink for the 'girls'. There was a bath on the female side but not on the male side. When I was admitted there were more women than men as patients, so the lower male six-bedded unit was occupied by women. At the lower end was a sitting room with TV and small library connected to a dining area. From this was a door that gave access to a small enclosed patio garden. At the top end of the ward by the entrance there were a number of rooms, including those for doctors, senior nurses, kitchen, storage, and a larger room for general use, including patient activities such as painting etc. The well-equipped physio-therapy and occupational area was a short distance away along the entrance corridor.

I was initially put into a bed in the upper male six-bed ward and was 'welcomed' by the nurse on duty, who also arranged for me to get a sandwich, since it was by now after the ward lunch-time. The rest of that first day was a blur, which meant that it passed quickly and I slept reasonably well overnight, though it was noisy – both because of other patients and also the night staff, who chattered periodically.

The next morning I was asked by the nurse in charge if I would like to change to the single room, as this was going to become available. With little doubt, I said, 'Yes, of course.' This was a decision which was to prove an important and extremely critical one for me. That morning I was duly transferred to the single room, where I remained until I was discharged home in November.

The single room was spacious, and I saw that if necessary another bed could be put in. The adjacent room had in fact got two beds and patients in it. I noted with some pleasure that there was a TV on the wall, a channel changer for me to use, but only four channels – BBC 1, BBC 2, ITV and Channel 4 – perhaps I was looking for too much! There was a side cabinet for my use, a mobile tray table which could come over the bed, a tallboy for storage of clothes etc., a small washbasin, and a stunning view through a large window to the outside world. This encompassed a grassy bank, beautiful trees and shrubs, a bird feeder, and the main road exiting the hospital. Additionally, I had the call buzzer, together with controls for the bed height and positions, which was on a control panel attached by a cable to the wall behind the bed. Unlike ward 55, there was no hospital radio service on offer. Moira agreed that my room was very comfortable, and it was much more private than being in the general six-bedded area. The only downside was that it proved to be very hot when the sun shone in; the radiators were on 'winter setting', and for the first month I still suffered from sweating, night and day. A suitable fan was given to me for use as necessary.

The next thing on the agenda was to settle down and learn about the daily routine.

As time went by I became increasingly familiar with what was a reassuring process in many aspects. I usually awoke at about 6.30 a.m. just before the day staff came on duty at about 7 a.m. Presumably, there was a changeover exchange of information with the night staff before ward work began between 7.30 and 8 a.m. Some staff came in slightly later at 8 a.m. and some only worked until about 2 p.m. The rest worked through the day until about 7 p.m. when the new night staff came on duty and were apprised regarding the patients in the way of a report. At about 7.30 a.m. my jug of water was emptied and replenished with fresh water, and I turned the TV on to see the news programmes. Then, depending on the timetable for morning physiotherapy, I was either bed-bathed, bathed at side of my bed at the washbasin on my wheelchair, or taken down the corridor to be showered – this process tended to be done after breakfast if there was no physiotherapy that day, or at the weekends, when there was no physiotherapy. Breakfast was served by the nurses at about 9 a.m. and consisted of a cereal (Weetabix, porridge, or All-Bran flakes) and toast, which was as often colder than not! If I asked nicely I could often get warmer toast. Just before this, a separate nurse came and gave me my tablets, which were locked in the top drawer of my bedside cabinet. Further tablet distribution occurred at tea time (5 p.m.) and bedtime (10 p.m.).

Physiotherapy was usually a twenty to thirty-minute session, either in the morning or less often in the early afternoon. If I did not have physiotherapy, I filled in my time watching TV, reading, drawing and painting, watching DVDs, talking to visitors, using my PC, or resting... I felt surprisingly tired after visitors or physiotherapy sessions! Visitors, of whom there were many, usually came at the recognised visiting times between 3 and 4.30 p.m. and 6.30–8 p.m.

I could have lunch or tea in my room, or be taken down on my personal wheelchair to the sitting room where I could meet and talk with others. Lunch was at 12 p.m. and tea at 5 p.m., though fewer people went down for tea. One day per week, on either the male side or the female side, all those who could be moved to the sitting room were taken from their rooms or ward in order that a proper cleaning could be undertaken; as far as I could tell this was meticulously done each week. Hand antibacterial creams for visitors and staff were available in the rooms and ward areas. The meals were served by the nurses, and those patients who required help were assisted with feeding etc. (More on the food later!) 'Lights out' in the evening was done by the night nurses at about 10 p.m., but I was fortunate because in my own room I could watch the TV for a later time if I wished. A cup of tea and a biscuit was served by a tea lady mid-morning, mid-afternoon, and also in the evening. Each day, random blood pressure measurements and finger-prick blood-sugar measurements were usually done by the nurses and recorded in my records. The 'ward round' by the Professor was due each Thursday afternoon, but otherwise doctors were scarcely seen.

There were various events that occurred during the week and involved the help of a splendid group of 'volunteers'. These included quizzes, bingo, parties with afternoon teas, and other activities, usually on Tuesday evening; these it was interesting to see were attended by some senior boys and girls from local schools, including Daniel Stewart's College, Mary Erskine School for girls, and Edinburgh Academy. These enthusiastic young people served meals and helped, and were a credit to their schools as well as giving pleasure to the patients There were of course more senior lady volunteers, who were the main organisers and did additional things including the art clubs, visits outside to shops or other venues, as well as simply visiting to the patients to chat and so on. I consider these ladies to have contributed greatly to my care and the other patients. They were helped by the enthusiastic contribution made by Dr Elaine – the medical assistant of the Stroke Unit. Her personality and ideas brought increased stimulation for everyone.

The night-time staff introduced themselves at about 10 p.m. They provided urinary bottles as required, and tucked me in. Initially, this involved me being lifted up the bed and turned onto my left side, as I could not do this by myself. The sweating problem previously mentioned persisted for about six weeks initially, and the fan was frequently required. Should I require it to be turned off, or I needed to alter my position in bed, I pressed the buzzer to call for assistance. After about two months I found I was able to do these things myself. I only had to seek advice at night from a doctor on one occasion when I had a severe pain in the haematoma in my right groin which was settled by an analgesic; it was reassuring to know that a doctor was always 'on call' at night, and presumably during the day if required.

The Nurses and Doctors

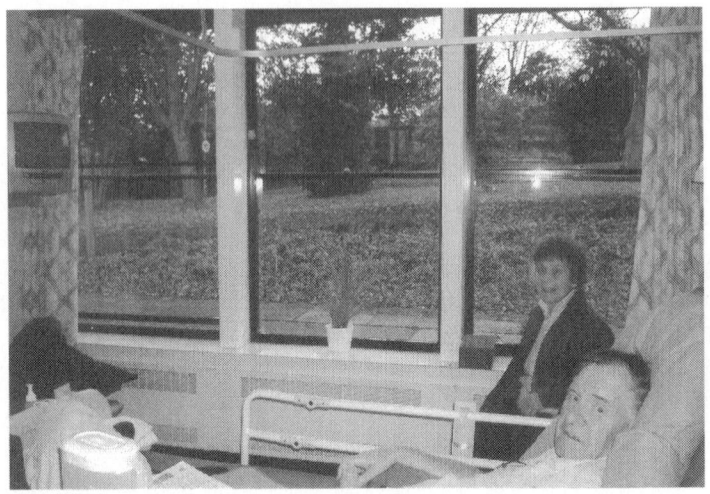

Photograph of my room and the view outside. Courtesy of Mr Alf Cattenach

This may be one of the shorter chapters, but that does not reflect on the significance and importance of this stage in my care and recovery. Having said this, I was in a good position to observe as a patient rather than a doctor who had worked for many years in the NHS as well as in the private scene, and as a surgeon rather than a physician.

As far as I could see, the nurses on each shift consisted of about three on the male side and presumably a similar number on the female side. Though the two groups did not necessarily mix during each shift, they did share if required, and of course might be on the other side the next shift. At night the same sort of distribution seemed to occur, and some of the day nurses had sessions at night. The reverse did not, to my knowledge, happen so often. Usually the nurses did not do more than two or three shifts at a time before being off duty for a few days. The more antisocial night-time shifts seemed to suit those who did them, and from what I could see they were less physically demanding. Quite often I heard the night staff talking loudly, and not always because of patient-related activities! Since I was in my own room and not in the ward areas I did not find this to be a major source of disturbance and I could also have my door shut. Using my buzzer at night usually resulted in a nurse coming promptly; the same could not be said during the day!

According to what I learned from the nurses, there was always a shortage, day and night, and accordingly 'bank nurses' were called on to help almost every day! This agreed with my observations during my stay. It was probable that about 30% of the nurses were 'bank nurses'. Some were extremely good, but it was not always reassuring to learn what one such nurse told me, that he/she had not worked in the stroke unit for many months, or did not know how apparatus worked or where everything was to be found! I learned from other patients that this was a constant concern and that some days were more of a worry because of unaccustomed staff. The staff also had their own worries with patients, and I was surprised to learn that some – and not just the black ones – had been subjected to racial and social abuse! (Occasionally this involved actual physical assault.)

Overall, the organisation and morale was excellent and this was to a great extent due to the outstanding leadership and example set by the senior nurses, led by the ward manager, Rachel. I found after a few weeks who were the really good nurses and who were not; the majority were hard working, very helpful, and understanding of the embarrassments and problems in a stroke patient. This was certainly something that I found invaluable on several occasions, not the least being the worrying dilemma I had when, owing to a troublesome and noisy ward patient, there had been a chance I would have to vacate my room for that person and be moved out into the six-bedded ward. A restless night of worry about this had ensued, but on hearing of my real concerns and dilemma about the move, Rachel quickly investigated the situation and solved the problem so that I stayed!

This was a great relief to me, and the patient received an appropriate solution that also solved the problem of disturbance in the ward for other patients. The majority of the nurses were female, but one of the best ones was male – a young man who had a real grasp of my problems and encouraged me to start to become more independent.

One thing I found somewhat strange to begin with was the tendency of the nurses to address me and the other patients using Christian names – probably because in my own work in hospital this was not usually the situation. As time went by I became adjusted to this – at least I was not called 'dearie' or 'darling'!

By way of contrast, the doctors were hardly in evidence, except for the periodic appearance during the weekdays when a junior doctor was needed for new admissions or some urgent patient need that could not be met by the nurses and Dr Elaine (Staff Grade doctor). Dr Elaine was also involved with the volunteers during the week and at other times in organising as well as taking active part in events and games for the patients. All of this was greatly appreciated, and as far as I am concerned was a very important part of the rehabilitation process; more about this in future chapters.

The Professor came once a week on Thursday afternoons and looked in to see me during this time. He seemed to me to be a man of few words and this, together with the fact there was no actual 'ward round' as I thought there might be was somewhat disturbing, if not disappointing. What I did not appreciate initially was that he and Dr Elaine had a meeting before they looked round the ward with representatives of the nurses, physiotherapists, and occupational therapists etc., and discussed their patients' management and progress.

Unfortunately, neither Moira nor I felt that feedback from these meetings was always forthcoming or relevant. Perhaps I was expecting too much; perhaps it was felt that since I was a doctor this was unnecessary. Certainly the time-honoured 'ward round' seems to be a relic of the past in both surgery and medical units. The absence of teaching of medical or postgraduate students seemed to be surprising, but perhaps I was considered 'out of bounds'. In fact I would have been happy to see them!

The Other Professional Therapists and the Volunteers

During my inpatient stay there were a number of other professionals who were involved in my care and to whom I am greatly indebted. At a very early stage in the stay in the Western Infirmary, I was seen by a therapist who assessed my ability to speak and another who assessed my abilities mentally. Both of these facilities seemed to me to be reassuringly normal. When I was transferred to the Royal Victoria Hospital, these examinations were repeated and developed. I was given a series of tongue exercises to practice, even though I did not think I had any speech disabilities, and a series of verbal tests to practise, including repeating tongue-twisters like 'The Leith police dismissal us'! After I had practised these for a few days I had to demonstrate to the therapist what I could do. I passed this test easily and was judged not to have any problems. I required no further treatment or assessment. The assessment of my mental status also involved a large number of questions, not rehearsed. The questions ranged from the basic 'who was I?', 'what is the day of the week?', 'where was I?' to more involved ones such as 'what would I use to drink tea out of?' or 'name as many animals as I can in ten seconds'! Needless to say it was decided fairly early on that I was completely normal for these tests also!

During August I had to go to the urology clinic in the Western General to investigate my bladder because of an episode of bloodstained urine which, though it was thought to be the result of infection, gave me some concern. As a result, it was found that I had an infection and a bladder with poor muscle tone, and this required a catheter for at least a further one month. After what turned out to be a long and tiring day, I returned to my room in the Royal Victoria with a new catheter strapped to my thigh and a prescription for more tablets! I was relieved at least that no serious tumour problem had been found, and there was the added advantage of less worry about using bottles etc. for a few more weeks!

The physiotherapists and the occupational therapists were of the greatest importance in my rehabilitation and were present throughout my inpatient stay, and with regard to afterwards, other physiotherapists continued the process when I got home.

I am not sure how often physiotherapy should be done for each patient, and presumably both amount and type depend on initial problems and progress, which would be different for every patient. What I had not taken account of was the fact that there is a national shortage of qualified physiotherapists – or rather, plenty of graduates but no money in the NHS to employ them! This situation had a bearing on my case, and when the senior physio-therapist who I saw initially in the first two days went off on long-term sick leave, she was not replaced and left the department short-staffed.

The remaining three girls, under Elizabeth, worked very hard none the less, and certainly did what they could. It appeared to me that they were stretched at times by the number of ward patients and consequently were not able to take patients either as often or for as long as they or the patients would have required. They did not of course work at weekends, so Saturdays and Sundays were 'free days'. Of the remaining five days of the week there was no guarantee that you would be taken on each day – as I found much to my disappointment. I was never taken every day; it was rarely four, and most commonly three days, and for times of about thirty minutes per session. It was true that to begin with my condition and easy tiredness probably merited only short and less frequent sessions, but this was not the case in the later months. In addition, I agreed to take part in a research project with the physiotherapists. This involved using a treadmill, on which I was supported on a series of slings for the first six weeks, and I was happy to participate, but it meant there was no extra time for extra physiotherapy sessions.

Whether this affected my result or progress remains uncertain but I was quite happy to be involved in what might yet prove to be a helpful addition to the care of suitable stroke patients. The fact that I had been selected as being suitable for this trial acted as a very positive 'plus' sign as far as I was concerned, and suggested that there was an expectation that one day I would be able to walk. Near the end of my inpatient physiotherapy the girls obtained additional help from an excellent senior student, who was due to qualify in less than one month; but told me she had 'no job' and also none to apply for – a situation apparently not uncommon for graduates like her, even given the apparent national shortage of physiotherapists! Surely this cannot be right?

The role of the physiotherapists in the care of strokes is vital and in my case was very important. Firstly, I considered that I was still relatively young and had both mental and vocal faculties intact, and secondly, I was highly motivated. My main objective was to be able to walk before I went home and accepted the opinion given to me at an early stage that the function of the right hand and upper limb would take longer and the outcome would in any event be unpredictable. At the outset I was able to sit comfortably on a bench or 'plinth' as it was termed. The next step over these early weeks was to try and stand up from the sitting position – not easy to begin with, but when achieved it enabled me to be transferred from bed to wheelchair to toilet or to the physiotherapy department. This was accomplished using a special intermediate device on wheels on which I stepped and was moved on wheels to the site of transfer firstly by means of an 'Encore' apparatus, which also lifted you into a standing position and, when I was able to stand up by myself, by a less bulky Samhall Turner transporter. This represented a major advance over methods using the sling system.

At this stage (mid-August) I noticed definite muscle activities returning in the front of my thigh and this greatly encouraged me. By now I was into the treadmill experiment, which may or may not have speeded up this improvement. The sole of my foot and the toes had normal sensation and proprioception, and though my foot was swollen and turned inwards because of muscle weakness this did not prevent me from standing for up to a minute at a time. The next stage was to try and take a step forward with support from the physiotherapists or by holding on to the plinth (whose height could be adjusted). This situation persisted for several weeks, but by the end of September I was able to walk slowly sideways around and holding on to the plinth. At this time also I noted that I could move my right middle finger!

It was during October that a major step forward took place, so to speak! I was now given the chance of taking a few steps, first supported, then on my own without anything. This was a truly wonderful experience, which was matched when a week later I walked the ten metres that was a standard that had to be achieved before being considered for being allowed home. Of course, getting home permanently had not yet been discussed, but I felt that it was getting nearer. I used the remaining three weeks that I stayed in the Royal Victoria improving my walking, and since I now had this increased freedom I was able to move about in my room and visit the toilet more easily. For the first time latterly I received some exercises to try and improve hand and arm function but compared to the recovery in my lower limb this seemed very poor and in particular my shoulder was stiff, immobile and painful.

The occupational therapists were also thin on the ground, and since a lot of their work involved visits to assess homes and advice on any modifications that were required before discharge home, ward visits were less frequent than was ideal. As far as I was concerned, they were a vital part of the team. They went to my home and advised on modifications such as rails on doors, walls and stairs etc., and when I went home finally they came and checked that I could get in through the front door, climb the stairs to my bedroom, get into and out of my bed, and get into and out of the bath using an easily mastered lifting frame. All of this closely involved Moira, of course, for without her it would have been less easy, if not impossible. The ward visits were infrequent but were just enough for me to get to know them and to be taught how to wash at the washbasin and to dress myself. The only things I found impossible to do unassisted were putting on my socks and shoes. Another important function they performed was to check that I could transfer from my wheelchair into a car seat and back into the chair. This would mean the end of uncomfortable wheelchair/taxi transfers.

One person who also came to see me once per week, although it was only in the last two months of my stay in hospital, was the aromatherapist. She only went to some patients – I am not sure why or how it was decided upon. I found the half-hour sessions to be most restful and enjoyable. Basically, she applied fragrant smelling ointment to my right foot, leg, and right shoulder and carefully massaged these areas. Whether it actually improved movements in these areas was difficult to say, but the mere fact of her coming in to see me and talk to me, together with the massage and nice fresh odours, did a great deal in making my stay more enjoyable.

Other people who came in and made life more enjoyable were the tea ladies, the water jug changer and room cleaner and the various volunteers. The latter group included the Tuesday night school children already mentioned, a lady who brought her dog in to visit the patients, another who watered any plants in the rooms, and a group of lady volunteers who, in addition to coming in and talking to me, organised games, special teas, birthday parties, visits for some who wished to go to shops etc., activities like an art club, and fund-raising events to help pay for these activities and other things for the stroke unit. I was surprised to learn, for example, that all the wheelchairs in the unit for the patients and the payment for the aromatherapist to visit the patients were all paid for out of non-NHS funds raised by these volunteers. Surely this might be something the NHS should be paying for anyway! Even the dinner tables and chairs in the patients' meal and recreation area were, I think, also supplied by volunteer donations.

As far as I am concerned, the role of the volunteers in helping me to recover was extremely important, and none more so than those I met through my introduction to the art club – more on this later.

Cards, Gifts and Visitors

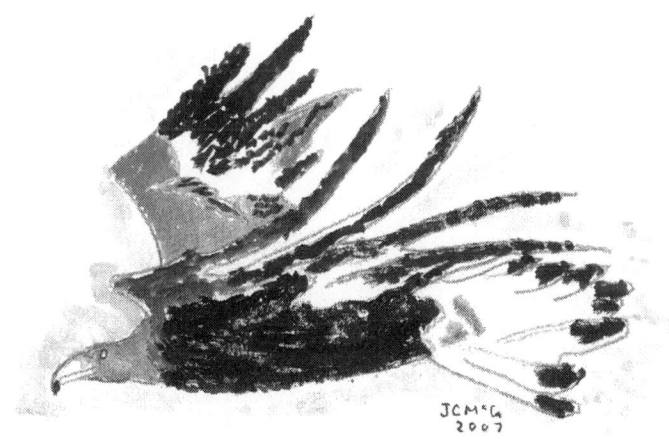

Painting of a flying eagle – one of my first efforts!

I received an embarrassing but very welcome number of 'get well' cards! The board above my bed could not take them all, and some went back with Moira to our home. Some came when I was home in late November and some came later in Christmas cards. They all meant a lot to me and helped to make me feel good. Some of the cards were from relatives, some from nurses and staff at the hospitals, some from my former colleagues, some from grateful patients, and some from friends. In many cases the cards had encouraging comments, and a few were extremely humorous and amused me greatly. It showed that I still had a good sense of humour!

Accompanying gifts were sent too, notably bouquets of flowers from the Secretariat of the British Association of Plastic and Aesthetic Surgeons, from the husband and wife of one of my previous consultant plastic surgery colleagues in St John's Hospital, West Lothian, the manager of Murrayfield Hospital, and another from a group of friends known as 'the Rugby Crowd' – more of them later. I received several bowls of delicious fruit from friends and a large basket from the theatre staff of Murrayfield Hospital. The staff of my former plastic surgery ward in St John's Hospital sent to my home two large garden shrubs, both beautifully presented and in pots. Two potted flowering plants that were able to grace my room window ledge were kindly given to me – one from a neighbour and the other from Mr Pradip Datta, who was a member of the Council of the Royal College of Surgeons of Edinburgh and outgoing honorary secretary. He delivered this personally and conveyed the best wishes of the College to me; I am a member of this College.

I was also fortunate in having a great number of visitors, though to begin with, while welcome, I found them quite tiring. As I began to get stronger and more mobile in my bed, visitors became less of a worry! The most consistent and loyal visitor was Moira, who I think only missed one day due to sickness and came twice a day throughout! She gave me great support during this worrying time and brought extra 'goodies' for me to eat, such as fruit and sandwiches, which were a very welcome supplement to what was becoming, as the months went by, a less appetising hospital meal service. I was visited by my cousin, Lynne, and husband, Alan, brothers-in-law and sisters-in-law, Ron and Edna, and Norman and Sheila.

Visitations by my daughter, Trudy, her husband, Andrew, and our grandchildren, Callum and Holly, greatly helped my spirits, as did my son Alan, daughter-in-law, Susanna, and grandson, Joshua, who came on holiday from India during August. A comment by son gave me great encouragement as well as illustrating our family spirit and sense of humour. It was, 'Dad, I am sure you will walk before your two youngest grandchildren [Holly and Joshua].' This proved to be true!

Although I have not been an avid churchgoer, I was very impressed by the frequent visitations by the Reverend Dr Russell Barr, minister of Cramond Church, his deputies, and our church elder, Mr Kenneth Archibald.

Other visitors of note included my old friend, Alisdair, a GP, who was best man at our wedding; he travelled down by motorbike from his home in Blairgowrie. Then there were two former Plastic Surgical Consultant colleagues from St John's, Awf Quaba and Stuart Hamilton; two representatives of the Edinburgh College of Surgeons, including Mr Pradip Datta; Catriona, of BUPA Murrayfield Hospital, Edinburgh; my Sunday morning golf partners, Niall, Eric and Findlay; and last but not least, my main anaesthetist at the latter hospital who came on several occasions, Dr David Brown.

What about 'the Rugby Crowd'? This is a group of our close friends who have been such from the school days of our sons, and they followed our boys playing rugby from primary school to when they left Daniel Stewart's College and thereafter. We have continued until the present day watching rugby at home and abroad, enjoyed holidays at home and overseas, had birthday and other parties together, and encouraged each other at times of stress and difficulties. This unique group – Ros and Phil, Meryl and Alf, Freda and Allan, John and Lesley, Eleanor and Alistair, and Jacqui – visited regularly and gave both Moira and myself great support and help in a major way. I am really most indebted to them.

There were a few surprises from people who either did not send cards or visit, but this might have been they did not know about my illness or felt it might have been embarrassing to see me 'with a stroke' – assuming that I might be embarrassed, and might not be able to speak and have a twisted face! There were on the other hand some surprise visitors and letters from unexpected sources.

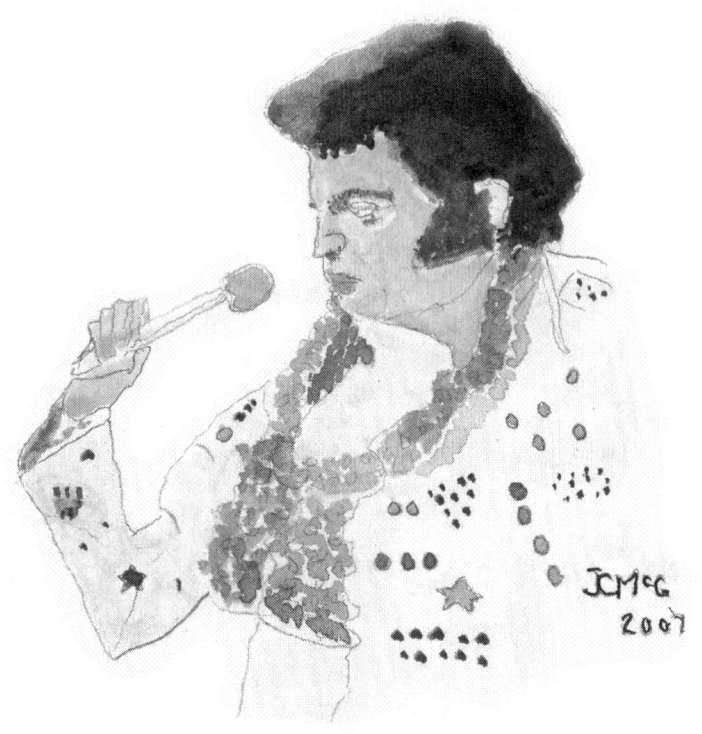

Elvis

How Did I 'Amuse' Myself?

One of the problems that may face all stroke patients is how to occupy themselves during what may be a stay in the ward for periods of up to, and occasionally more than, a year. In my case, possibly because of the type of stroke, the good progress I made, and my home circumstances, I was only in ward 9 for about 3½ months. Furthermore, I had no speech impairment or brain deficit affecting my thought processes. In other words I was fortunate in most aspects, not the least being that throughout my stay I was fortunate to have a large single room, a TV, and a nice view through large windows of the woodland and garden areas outside. The periods available for 'recreation' were those without physiotherapy or occupational therapy sessions, visiting times, and meals. This could be as much as three hours on weekday mornings, two hours in the weekday afternoons, and a further two or so hours in the evenings. More time was available at weekends when there was very little to do. I decided at the beginning that I would try to keep occupied as much as possible, believing that this would also help my recovery.

A. Games

The only game I used for a very short time was 'Pocket Sudoku', which came as a series of magnetic pieces in a tin board and was, as far as I was concerned, beyond me to solve, though very easy to handle in the bed and with only one hand. A major problem was that it sometimes slipped onto the floor, spilling all the tiny letters! In my view, had I been an expert or keen sudoku player I think this game would have been very useful.

B. Books etc.

At a very early stage I was given a book written by Robert McCrum entitled *My Year Off* – about his harrowing yet rewarding experience and recovery from a severe stroke. This, in fact, did help me to understand more about a stroke, and the story about his slow but steady and remarkable recovery should be an inspiration to all – I thoroughly recommend it!

I also continued my attempt at learning Spanish using a small language book (*Teach Yourself Instant Spanish* by Elisabeth Smith) and can recommend for easy and interesting reading a small book by New Scientist entitled *Why Don't Penguins' Feet Freeze? and 114 Other Questions*, edited by Mick O'Hare. I also subscribed to a new magazine called *Wildlife of Britain*, which is produced in easily read form and illustrated with beautiful pictures.

Moira brought in some daily papers to read and I tried my best to turn the pages but found this difficult with only one 'good' hand. For some unknown reason, daily papers were delivered to some ward patients but not me!

C. DVDs

The portable DVD apparatus given to me by Alan was easily plugged in, and over the duration of my stay proved to be a wonderful accompaniment. Prior to my stroke I had collected a large series of Sir David Attenborough's wild life TV series and steadily worked my way through these with wonder and great enjoyment. Some of the images in these are truly outstanding. The other thing that I greatly enjoyed was using it for music – not classical! Perhaps, this readership and my friends will be surprised to learn that I 'rocked' in my wheelchair and bed to Queen, Elvis Presley and Elton John. All that was missing were Motown artists, Bon Jovi, and Tina Turner! None of my searchers could locate these during my stay. I felt that this stimulating music, which I have always enjoyed, would keep my spirits up and possibly stimulate brain cell recovery, though I had no strong evidence for this latter view.

D. The TV

Although there were only four channels available – BBC 1, BBC 2, ITV and Channel 4 – this was 'heaven' for me, and with a channel changer at my bedside, it gave me the feeling of power as well as freedom. I could watch what I liked, when I liked, and did not need to refer to anyone else. It did not matter to me that there was no hospital radio service, as there had been in the Western General, but this would have been an additional bonus, especially when the TV programmes on offer were no good to me. I liked the news and documentary programmes best of all, and the sport. I enjoyed the nature programmes, especially *Autumnwatch* and found to my surprise that I became 'interested' in the *Jeremy Kyle Show*, where unbelievable and difficult social problems were exhibited and discussed openly with members of the public. I found myself watching other programmes that I would not normally have watched – some of which annoyed me greatly. In this category I would include the large number of cooking programmes with celebrity chefs, the selling and makeover of houses, and the frivolous 'shows' like *Loose Women*. Other programmes that I liked included *Dragons' Den*, *Holby City*, *Richard and Judy*, *Antiques Roadshow*, and *EastEnders*.

E. The Personal Computer

My computer could also be easily be brought in and plugged in at my bedside, and this gave me a further possibility for useful activities. One of my interests includes writing, and over the years I have written and had quite a lot of work published in various medical journals. I was keen to continue this if possible, and my illness stimulated my thought processes and also, with time on my hands so to speak, it seemed a good idea to pursue this. While I was not able to use my right hand, it was really not difficult to use the computer. Two articles were completed and accepted for publication in the Edinburgh College of Surgeons production, *Surgeons' News*.

The first article related to the importance of a 'name', and how the name we are given at birth may affect our career or success in life. This was developed into the various ways available to us to investigate our own relatives and forebears including the new method using DNA analysis. The second article was on the subject of 'left-handedness', and discussed the incidence under normal circumstances and whether or not any special advantages were conferred. The question as to whether left-handed persons were more artistic was posited and, if, as in my case, it could explain my apparent abilities to use my left hand (though previously being right-handed). The acceptance of these articles and their preparation gave me considerable satisfaction.

F. Views out of my window and surroundings

Not only did I have a single room but I also had an excellent view outside to look at through the long days. This scene included a bird feeder pole that had hanging baskets and sometimes a half-coconut. As far as I could ascertain, it was visitors who filled up the feeders with bought bird food – usually peanuts. Surprisingly, but probably because there was no anti-squirrel devices, I saw very few small birds such as blue tits at this feeder. The main visitors were a pair of grey squirrels, who seemed to frighten everything else away; but in the months of August and September two wood pigeons were a match for them at ground level. These pigeons were sometimes accompanied by a strange-looking friend – possibly a juvenile bird – and stopped coming in October when autumn leaves had started to fall. Other visitors around the feeding area were two common crows, a number of magpies, some tiny field mice, and various cats – the latter to be seen clearly stalking and catching mice. On some occasions I saw up to a dozen squirrels or magpies cavorting about the feeder and surrounding woodland. All of these antics helped me to feel more relaxed as well as making my days more interesting. During the night-time, although the curtains were closed, I enjoyed hearing the sounds of tawny owls screeching and, in the dawn, the sounds of wrens, robins, and even the noisy crows. Strangely I never saw blackbirds, robins, or thrushes near the feeder. Seagulls some-times came down to eat food thrown out of a window by a patient!

The total scene visible from my room was only part of the greater woodlands and gardens surrounding the hospital. These, with their paths and enclosed gardens, offer a restful ambiance for the patients, visitors, and staff, one which the other hospitals such as the Western General or new Royal Infirmary in Edinburgh cannot offer. In the past, gardeners had been employed to keep these areas in good order but, owing no doubt to lack of NHS finance, this was no longer done to the same degree – in other words these areas had become a little 'overgrown' and neglected.

In front of my window there was a paved path along which hospital staff came and went, and some of them smiled at me as they got to recognise me. I found this to be something that kept me in touch with the outside world! In front of the path was a grassy bank, above which was a larger area of meadows containing some shrubs and trees. The bird feeder was situated in the grassy bank. Above the meadow runs the main exit road for the hospital, which was supposed to be one-way and to have a speed limit of 10 mph! It was interesting to watch the traffic and how often these restrictions were ignored!

The sun moved from left to right through each day, becoming lower as the winter months approached and forming beautiful colours and patterns through the trees. When autumn arrived and the leaves started to fall, the grassy meadow became covered with a brown/red carpet which provided a restful and colourful scene which changed from day to day and was made to 'dance' when the autumnal winds caused the leaves to dance around in mini-tornados.

G. *The role of the Volunteers and other patients*

The important role of the lady volunteers has already been mentioned before, but more needs to be said. Several were involved, giving up their time during the day and some evenings during the week; I believe that Elaine, Jennie, and Kay were the main organisers helped by the enthusiastic Dr Elaine. Various patient-oriented entertainments were organised, including games of bingo, dominoes, and quizzes, special afternoon teas, fish and chip suppers, music nights etc. I can remember especially one such evening of musical entertainment involving a talented entertainer who had come down from Blairgowrie. The entertainments were not limited to in-house activities, and during my stay some were taken out one evening to see the Edinburgh

Military Tattoo. I myself and one other wheelchair patient, David, were taken out to two Rugby Internationals at Murrayfield Stadium in the autumn, which were really enjoyable even though both games were won by the opposition – New Zealand and South Africa (who went on to win the Rugby World Cup later that year.) A surprise visit by Doddie Weir, the famous former Scottish international, to have a chat, a bite to eat, and share a small 'dram' after the first match in the 'social' room in ward 9, was really appreciated and enjoyed. It says a great deal about Doddie that he took the time to come out of his way to come and see us.

The real find for me with regard to the work of the volunteers came totally unexpectedly when I joined, at their invitation, the art club, which was held once or twice a week in the 'social' room. I was given a pencil and several books to look at with a view of trying to draw using my unaffected hand – something I had never tried before! The results were quite good and caused a reasonable amount of praise. I was encouraged to continue with art and consider watercolour painting, again something I never previously tried. I was given a drawing pad, a brush, and a dish of paint pigments. Thereafter I was 'off', and spent part of every day drawing and painting, encouraged by positive comments by others, and continued throughout my stay to do this very relaxing pastime. I was particularly pleased when some of my efforts were made into gift or Christmas cards for sale at the ward entrance to raise funds for the stroke unit. One of these – a smiling snowman – proved to be a very popular card at Christmas time, and raised a lot of money. If there is anything that raised my spirits most of all during my hospitalisation and revealed 'my hidden self', it was the art club.

I got to know some of the patients largely through the social events, but also through going down to the ward lounge for lunch or tea when, in our various chairs, wheeled or otherwise, we were sat around wooden tables. The meals were served by our ward nurses from a mobile electrically heated container. There were always three courses – a starter (usually soup), a choice of hot middle course, and a sweet (usually custard, ice cream, jelly, sponge, or rice pudding). Some patients were not fit enough to come for meals and stayed in their beds, and, though there were more women patients, there were always more men who came for meals; I never found out why this should be. The nurses helped those who for various reasons were unable to eat by themselves and gently encouraged those who did not seem keen to eat. A few patients seemed to me to eat very little, but I learned subsequently that their relatives or friends brought in sandwiches, etc. and this was not discouraged.

As far as I could understand, and much to my surprise, none of the meals were prepared on site, but actually had been prepared far away in Wales! The general opinion of the patients I spoke with was that the food was 'reasonable,' but this view altered the longer they stayed in! I must say that this became my view, and towards the end of my own sojourn I found the lack of variety, the odours of the cooked foods, and the poor taste was definitely a turn-off! Fortunately, Moira kept me well – but not too well – fed!

I was struck by the variety of ages among the patients as well as the different of types of stroke and their effects. Some were younger than me, some could not speak at all or with difficulty, some could not walk, some seemed very withdrawn, weepy and depressed, while some were much more upbeat and positive in their attitudes. I was particularly moved by the young woman who had been admitted for about a year and was unable to talk or walk initially, and who was discharged a month or so before me, ambulant with a stick and able to talk. At the other end of the scale was a ninety-year-old totally blind retired surgeon who had trained in Edinburgh but spent much of his life working abroad in China and India, and who was wheelchair bound. He had to be helped with almost everything, including being fed, and was always cheerful and uncomplaining.

I got to know some patients very well, but they were generally those who were able to communicate and discuss things of mutual interest. My being a doctor did not affect this, and I seemed to be accepted by them as another 'patient'. Also, possibly, being a doctor with no special 'image' problem, I was able to understand and talk with all types of patients. The difficulties discussed included worries about their jobs, driving cars again, lack of relatives, including spouses, to help, the food in the hospital, going home, delays in getting home/modifications that had to be done so they could get home, the infrequency or general lack of physiotherapy given, and comments about the nursing staff and care – not all of which was complimentary. Several comments related to 'rudeness' and embarrassment at toilet or bath times, but in general this was not a universal complaint and the nursing staff were often or not, highly praised.

For my part I consider that the ability to meet and interact with fellow patients to have been a most useful exercise, and that it can go a long way in aiding progress and understanding of the stroke and its effects.

My Progress from Admission to Ward 9 until my Discharge Home in November 2007

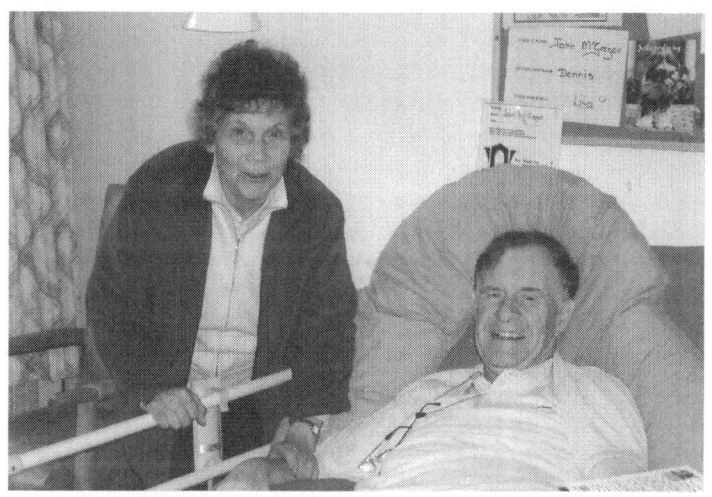

Photograph of Moira and myself near to the day of discharge from ward 9. Courtesy of Mr Alf Cattenach

The fact that I was only in hospital for about four months, and about three months and two weeks in the Royal Victoria Hospital, was due to a number of factors including my own determination, the type of stroke, my home circumstances, my wife, and the progress I made with what can be termed 'transfer and mobility issues'. Obviously, when some of these were not ideal, there could be delays in some patients' cases, and I saw this in the unit. Although I have been critical of my physiotherapy and the therapists' occupational therapy, I have to admit by the time I was discharged, I was able to stand up, walk with a stick, get up stairs, and get in and out of bed and bath. They suggested suitable modifications related to fitting of rails at the front door and upstairs landing, an extra banister on the stairs, and an easily used bath lift. These were quickly and easily fitted in and all of it was free! Moira had also purchased an electric wheelchair and also a lightweight, hand-pushable wheelchair, together with a ramp, which would help these over the small front doorstep in our house.

When I was first admitted to ward 9, I had no significant movement in my right hand or upper limb apart from a tiny flicker on the side of my middle finger and a definite muscle activity in my right thigh (medial quadriceps). Transfer to and from the bed to wheelchair and to the toilet, to meals in the lounge, or for physiotherapy, was done with the help of the nursing staff and the standing frames on wheels already mentioned. Thank goodness there was no need to use the slings and more elaborate devices in my case, although I saw their use for some of the other patients.

Towards the end of August I was able to walk a few steps with support from physiotherapists or other helpers, including Moira, and this enabled me to go out to the Cramond Church for my granddaughter Holly's christening, and to a buffet lunch at the Royal Burgess Golf Club using a taxi that took the wheelchair. This was my first real venture outside, and though tiring was a great experience and paved the way for the next stage in my recovery – a number of short weekend day visits to my home. Moira made sure I was comfortable and safe, together with the provision of refreshing meals; I was returned safely by taxi to ward 9 each evening. On 23 September, Dr Elaine and one of the ward nurses took me and another patient by taxi and wheelchair to Murrayfield Stadium to see New Zealand playing Scotland at rugby. A wonderful day was had by all, with an excellent view of the match from the disabled stance in the West Stand, spoiled by a Scotland defeat, but made even more enjoyable by meeting Doddie Weir later that evening. Three weeks later I was taken by car by Dr Elaine to another match at Murrayfield – Scotland versus South Africa. Prior to this I had demonstrated to the physiotherapists satisfactory transfer ability from wheelchair into and out of a car. Again, a great day for me, but Scotland still lost!

The result of the new transfer possibility was that no longer did my home visits need to be by taxi, as Moira could use our car. This was much easier as well as more convenient.

At this time I was steadily getting better at walking, firstly holding on to the plinth and going around the four sides, then a few steps with assistance of the physiotherapists, then a few steps on my own, and then, in the last month, I walked the ten-metre test distance advocated before consideration of getting home. Simultaneously, and even before this, the occupational therapists had ensured that I could perform basic washing at the room handbasin, shave myself with a battery-powered shaver, and put on some clothes. The putting on of socks and shoes remained a problem for me, however. To help with a tendency for my right foot to drag on walking, I was fitted with a special foot/ankle splint, which made it easier to move forward.

Moira was once again of great assistance and encouragement with regard to my mobilisation, both while I was in the hospital and also when increasingly I was allowed home at weekends. By the end of October I had been able to stay Friday night until Sunday evening at home, and slept in a bed brought downstairs. This, I found, was excellent preparation for eventual home-coming both for me and for Moira.

Jenny, a near neighbour and herself a physiotherapist, gave invaluable advice. She was careful, however, to not contradict or undermine the advice given by the ward 9 staff.

During the last three weeks there was no doubt that my impatience to get home markedly increased, as did my determination to improve my walking and independence in mobility in the wheelchair, such that I now felt confident to get to the toilet myself! There was also the great feeling when, almost to the applause of watching nurses and bed-bound patients, I was able to walk unassisted the complete distance of the corridor from my room down to the patient lounge and back! I had to be careful, though. Owing to my enthusiasm I had three times in the last month slipped off my wheelchair in my room, causing great concern amongst the nursing staff. Because of the noise this created, several of them arrived in far less time than any buzzer would have managed! Fortunately, no injury was sustained – only a few bruises to body and ego, a lecture, and worst of all – a notice on my cabinet which said bluntly, 'Fall risk'!

During this last period of time I was able to think about a number of philosophical issues, some of which arose through comments made by other patients and my visitors.

Most of my visitors said that I looked well, and probably this was true, although I did not always felt it to be the case. The comments included also that I had great 'motivation' and 'courage', and while these were very pleasing, I did not feel I was anything special. In my own personal experience over the years I have encountered many braver patients – young people with hideous deformities or tumours, a serious firework injury causing a major facial destruction and blindness, yet the man was able to return to lectures, etc. There was also a young lawyer who returned to a useful life in spite of loss of all four major limbs due to meningitis. With regard to strokes, there were plenty of examples of great personal recoveries, including those who were able to return to useful work and even drive modified cars. One such former patient visited me while I was at the art club and demonstrated this very fact. He had been able to return to his work as an architect after his severe stroke.

On television I was very interested to see a documentary on the bravery and return to active professional life as a pop star of Edwyn Collins, who had a hit record entitled 'A Girl Like You' in 1995, and who himself suffered a major haemorrhagic stroke in 2005, involving not only his limbs on one side but also his speech. Examples outwith strokes, and in which there are equally great bravery and survival in the face of great adversity, are not too difficult to find. They include the remarkable Stephen Hawking, who has a severe form of motor neurone disease and is only able to speak from a wheelchair by using a computerised voice production system.

Nor was my 'incarceration' in hospital for four months really such an ordeal, especially when compared to the ordeal of hostages like Terry Waite or Alan Johnston, who had been a hostage in Gaza over almost the same time as my stay. As Dr Elaine, herself a mother of several children, said to me on the day of my discharge home, I had only been an inpatient for four months 'which was only a small part of a full pregnancy'!

On my last day, I was given the opportunity of putting some of my observations on my stay and treatment in hospital to a representative of the Health Board (director of strategic planning and modernisation at NHS Lothian) who was visiting with Professor Dennis. Whether any of my observations and suggestions will be acted on remains to be seen, but my experiences while working in the NHS suggests that doctors' ideas are usually ignored.

My main conclusion was that the NHS was alive, and as far as I was concerned, and for my co-patients in the stroke unit, the care had been generally good. As far as I was concerned there are a number of issues, including a shortage of nurses (not bank or agency), a severe shortage of physiotherapists and occupational therapists, too much reliance on the nurses, rather than the doctors, to examine and communicate important clinical details to the patients and their relatives; and, from talking to the nurses, there was a lack of helpful support or even visitations from 'the administration staff' in the 'offices outside'. Before I left I presented the staff with a painting I had done inspired by my experiences and by a picture in a book I had seen at the art club. It was written by George Bruce with illustrations by Elizabeth Blackadder. Attached to a drawing of a dragonfly was an apt short verse or haiku.

> You brought my hidden
> Self into the light and it
> Was not at a loss.

Was I ready to go home? You bet I was!

Part Three

Home and What Happened until July 2008

Reflections and the First Three Months at Home

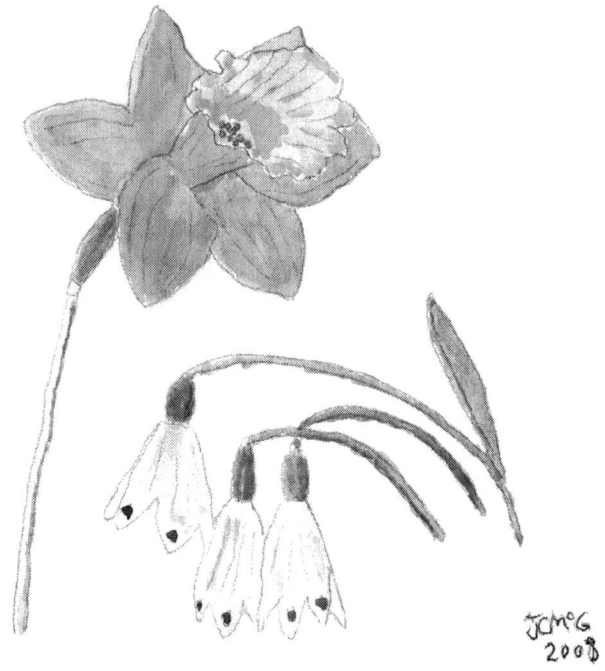

Painting of daffodil and snowdrops

There was no doubt that getting home was a wonderful experience, but for myself as well as Moira it was not without some worries about what was after all going to be a significant event. It transpired however that there would be much greater advice and help from the community than we had been lead to believe from the hospital. Perhaps we had not asked enough questions about this, but very little information was given out prior to my discharge.

The first thing I came to terms with fairly early on was that my operating days were over, no matter how good a recovery I could make with regard especially to my right hand. As I had decided prior to my stroke to retire either later in 2007, or at the latest in March 2008, this was not particularly a concern to me. I was disappointed that for some of my patients with problems I would not be able to complete surgery, but I was confident that my colleagues at Murrayfield Hospital would be able to advise and help; this has proved to be the case. I also was very content with my career in plastic surgery, it having been one that I chose to do while I was still at school, and, in spite of all the inherent difficulties, having proved to be a challenging and worthwhile choice. Indeed, it was one I felt extremely proud and privileged to have been involved in.

I also came to terms with the unlikelihood of pursuing in the immediate period my desire to travel to far off places, but since both my career and also a fondness for family holidays had enabled me to visit almost every continent in the world, this was not a major loss. For example, I have visited the Taj Mahal, walked on the Great Wall of China, viewed Cape Town from Table Mountain, have been on various safaris in Africa and seen the Victoria Falls, been to the Great Barrier Reef and Ayers Rock in Australia, been to see Las Vegas, the Grand Canyon, and Graceland, where Elvis lived, shopped with my wife in Hong Kong and Dubai, visited Jordan and Petra, managed to see the ancient ruins in Machu Picchu, been to Paris, Rome, Athens, Prague, Cyprus, Spain, Portugal, and Iceland, climbed the Statue of Liberty, viewed the beauties of Vancouver, and Western Canada, Toronto, the Niagara Falls, and Rio de Janeiro. I particularly enjoyed my teaching and examination duties, mostly arranged by the Edinburgh College of Surgeons, which took me to such places as Hong Kong, Chennai in India, Riyadh in Saudi, and Kuala Lumpur, and gave me the chance to see other cultures and hospitals. Outwith these, I had the great privilege of visiting Budapest, Bulawayo, and Curitiba in South America at the request of local plastic surgeons. The same degree of satisfaction and pleasure came to me from being, firstly an examiner, and more recently, an examiner of the examiners for the British Association of Plastic and Aesthetic Plastic Surgeons when I visited other British and Irish plastic surgery units. Finally, I have found great enjoyment in writing, and have to date published over one hundred articles in medical and associated journals, so I hoped to be able to continue writing! I was encouraged by a number of friends to consider writing a book on my experiences following my stroke, and after careful thought I decided to try this.

A real change in lifestyle was inevitable but some of this would have happened in any case when I retired and would involve me being more at home with my wife – a fact that neither Moira nor I had been particularly concerned about. The extra element now was that I had had an unexpected problem as the result of a stroke.

Many new problems were expected but we were both strong and determined to cope.

One of the first things to consider was my medication and my diet, neither of which I had needed to think about prior to my illness. With regard to my pills, these were needed to treat high blood pressure, diabetes, high cholesterol, reduce clotting, and some urinary problems that were possibly aggravated by a stroke. A total of ten tablets were prescribed to take each morning, two more at teatime, and a further two at bedtime! This requires great care each week, usually at the weekend, when Moira and I sat down and looked out the daily doses each day for the next week and put them into small plastic boxes which were obtained at the local chemist and called a 'mediMemo'. How an older person on their own would manage I do not know, and presumably there might be worries in case they took the wrong dose or forget altogether! With regard to diet this meant an end to crisps, fish and chips, fizzy drinks, and sugary or salty foods, all of which I admit I had indulged in before. There is at present much debate as to what would be a healthy diet for the general public, and much confusion regarding food content labelling and sugar, salt, fat, and calorie content. There was the additional fact that I was more at home than before, and more meals would have to be prepared. An excellent and not too expensive aid to help was found by using the Wiltshire Farm Food delivery service, which delivered every fourteen days a series of pre-ordered meals selected from their colourful brochure. These were stored in a freezer and when brought out were prepared finally in a micro-wave oven. By choosing from the brochure it was possible to ensure the products chosen were sugar-free, salt-free, low fat etc. Moira certainly felt that this was a very valuable service that made her life as a helper much easier.

I was delighted to be home yet felt a definite sense of frustra-tion that I was not as mobile as I had been prior to my stroke and had to rely on Moira much more – not that she complained, as she was pleased that I was home for good. What came next proved to be an unexpected surprise and help because it had only been discussed by an unknown man who came to ward 9 on the morning of my discharge. He had explained that he represented the Community Rehabilitation Service or CRS, which provided a service for people on discharge from hospital that would be tailored to the individual and his or her needs. In addition, a programme of activities could be arranged, including washing and dressing, exercise programmes, stair training, walking, shopping, social activities, and using public transport. This service is operated seven days a week but was only available for an initial period of five weeks. Once I was home, during the first week a representative of that service came to see me at home to discuss and arrange what should be done. It was decided that they would come twice daily on weekdays only, and concentrate on improv-ing my walking and the function of my right hand and arm with physiotherapy.

This was carried out by about six members of a team, includ-ing a physiotherapist, Dawn; an occupational therapist, Alison; and a rehabilitation worker, Kenny. Additionally, there was a visit from a stroke nurse, Sheila, who I never met while I was in the ward; she visited and discussed any problems that we had or anticipated. This nurse was officially the stroke nurse attached to ward 9, and her card indicated that her job was to 'offer inde-pendent, confidential advice, information and support to stroke patients and their families in the community'. As far as I can tell, these services are all part of a 'Managed Clinical Network' based in Edinburgh, but the service covers fifteen areas all over Scotland following the Scottish Parliament decision when it took over the NHS in Scotland. It is designed to improve the care of patients who have chronic illnesses such as heart disease, stroke, vascular disease, diabetes, and cancer. The 'Chest, heart, and stroke, Scotland' unit, which is part of this, aims to offer a range of community services throughout Scotland, including support for patients, families, and carers. This unexpected help certainly made me more comfortable, and I must admit I was completely surprised at the behind-the-scenes help and advice that was available to Moira as well as me.

Since I was now at home I received more visits from friends and neighbours and I was much more comfortable with this and less tired. I enjoyed their chat and comments – most would say with some apparent surprise how well I looked! This I accepted even though I still did not feel 100%! I was especially pleased as well as surprised by visitations from Alistair (best man) and Jessie, his wife; Eleanor and Moira (members of the organising committee of the Plastic Surgery Specialty examinations); retired consultants Dr Beveridge and Dr Smart; our church elder, Mr Archibald; my own relatives, including brothers and daughters-in-law; Niall, one of my golfing pals; and most important, my two Edinburgh-based grandchildren, Callum and Holly, who are a source of great pleasure and happiness. I would look forward to seeing my other grandson, Joshua, and his parents, due to visit us in March before their holiday abroad in Europe.

At an early time help was obtained which was to be very useful firstly in enabling me to get about more in the outside world and secondarily for Moira. This was the Disabled car sticker and a taxi card which made car parking and transportation using taxis use easier and a little less expensive. It was the case that I did not wish to go out too much to begin with until both the weather was warmer and I felt my mobility was better. Visits to see my GP, Dr Donald, and urology and diabetic clinics in the Western General Hospital were done before Christmas. All seemed to be progressing well with regard to my GP and diabetic control, but the urologist, Dr Tolley, was less pleased with some aspects. I would be attending more appointments in the New Year and expected to be assessed at the blood pressure clinic and also by Professor Dennis.

One of my first social visits outside was one at the request of the hospital volunteers to a lunch at the Caledonian Hotel in Edinburgh hosted by the Cruden Foundation, who were one of the providers of funds to be used by the volunteers, for purchase of patient wheelchairs, and payment to enable the aromatherapist to visit the ward patients etc. In return for my lunch (which was excellent) I gave a brief talk as a former patient, describing my experiences in the ward and how beneficial their contribution to me and the volunteers had been. Hopefully, this will be useful in securing their continuing interest! Other useful and morale-boosting outings early on were birthday parties for one of 'the Rugby Crowd' and for Callum and Holly (in January), and an invitation to be the chairman of a social holiday quiz for the plastic surgeons I had worked with at St John's Hospital. Christmas and New Year were relatively quiet periods, although Moira and I were treated to our Christmas lunch by Andrew and Trudy in their new house. Again, it was a most enjoyable outing for me.

At the end of January one of the boldest outings to date was undertaken to the Murrayfield Hospital Burns Supper held on the evening of the 26th in the George Hotel in Edinburgh. Here I was able to meet many of my former working nursing and medical colleagues. I survived this event unscathed and felt my confidence greatly enhanced by the experience. There were two visits for lunch with friends to the Bruntsfield golf club that I greatly enjoyed also.

The visits by the care/rehabilitation team were twice daily for a five-week period up to Christmas time. In the mornings, the work was usually regarding trying to improve the activity of my right hand and shoulder, which I must say had not received much attention before. Various exercises were given to me to practise in between their visits, and after their work had been completed, I did feel that some improvements were made in shoulder and finger movements. Greater improvements seemed to result from the afternoon sessions when, depending on the weather, I was taken outside for walking practice in the local streets. At this time I was still wearing the foot/ankle splint to reduce foot dragging, and I used a walking stick outside of our house. Subsequently I was referred to the Astley Ainslie Hospital in Edinburgh for fitting of an electrical nerve stimulator, which did the same job in a more physiological way, thereby dispensing with the need to wear the splint.

Under the regime of this initial five-week period, I certainly progressed with regard to my walking outside with the super-vision and accompaniment of the helpers and Moira, who also took me to the Gyle Shopping Centre. Initially, I was only able to walk on the outside pavements about fifty yards, but progressed to about twice that within a week or so. It was much easier to walk on the smoother surface indoors in the Gyle, and I only had to 'dodge' the other pedestrians and sometimes wheelchairs! On 11 January I walked the whole length of the Gyle Shopping Centre and doubled this distance the next day – timewise, this was done in about fifteen minutes. I progressed to being able to walk unaccompanied in our local streets, which of course freed Moira, as well as giving me more freedom and confidence. The weather was kind, and each day I was able to carefully increase the distances I was able to go and my stamina appeared to be increasing.

After the rehabilitation staff had completed their period of supervision I was very fortunate to be referred to the McLeod Street physiotherapy by my GP, Dr Donald. There I was to go once a week for an unspecified time to see a specialist stroke physiotherapist – Julie – who in fact had been highly recommended to Moira and myself by several hospital friends. Her advice, subsequent care, and exercise programmes were of fantastic benefit to me over the next period of time, both for my walking and for my hand and shoulder. On her advice, a special hand splint was obtained and fitted to try and reduce the periodic spasm I had causing 'locking' of my fingers. This was the 'SaeboStretch' splint. It was to be worn for intermittent periods of time during each day, and during the night if possible.

By the middle of February, Holly was able to stand and walk a few tottering steps and Joshua was crawling, as we saw on our webcam link with our family in Delhi. Thus I had been able to walk before them! I was now able to go out twice each day for increasing distances, depending on the weather. Whether due to 'global warming' or natural climatic variations, the winter – and February in particular – was proving to be surprisingly mild and sunny, and so this made walking in the immediate areas around our house very accessible for me as well as very pleasant. The only things that made things tricky were the periodic gusts of wind and the poor state of the pavements. While I had to watch carefully where I placed each step, I had 'time', as the famous golfer, Jack Nicklaus, once said, 'to smell the flowers'! At this period of the year, of course there were few odour-producing flowers, but there were white and pink winter heaths, purple autumn crocuses, and pure white snowdrops to enjoy visually in the gardens, where I could also listen to the birds that were singing at this time of year.

As a keen ornithologist from my boyhood, I now had more time than in my working life to listen and observe. A large flock of honking geese in typical 'V' formation flew high over the house from north to south one morning; I wondered where they had come from and where they were going! I watched for a few minutes a pair of long-tailed tits cavorting in a leafless bush and marvelled at their beauty and apparent oblivion to my presence – truly a magic moment! I listened to the sounds of the local bird population: the piping sounds of the great tits, the warbling territorial robins and hedge sparrows, the early beginnings of the chaffinches' and greenfinches' longer songs, a distant song thrush melody, the occasional house sparrow 'chirruping' from the depths of a beech hedge, a starling 'churring' from a rooftop TV mast, and the coarser outbursts of crows, magpies, or jackdaws. All of this was a truly wonderful experience for me during this period of my recuperation. Add to this the fresh air on my face and the new freedom in my life and you can probably empathise with my enthusiasm!

By now it was seven months since the onset of my illness and I had been out of hospital for three months. It had been a challenging period in my life. It would be interesting to see how much progress could be made in the next five months, which would bring me up to one year from my stroke.

"DAISY!"

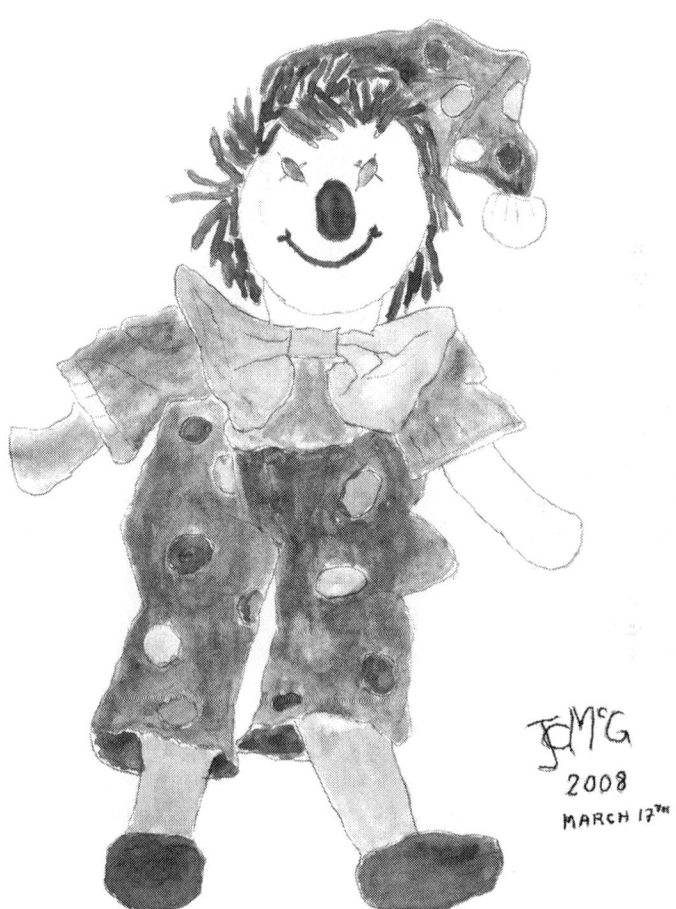

'Daisy', the neighbour's doll

The Following Five Months until July 2008 –
the Early Period

At this time it was just over halfway towards the full year after the stroke, and it was at the stage when I was beginning to see the light of day, so to speak! The days were beginning to lengthen, springlike activities just starting, and nature was becoming more evident. Since I was now able to get up and about more and felt stronger, my morale and desire to improve were in no doubt. I think this was also true for Moira, who was now more adjusted to my condition and was allowing me to do more things for myself. My aim at this stage was to continue with improvement and strive for more independence. I hoped to improve the function of my right hand and upper limb, be able to drive a car, be able to play golf to some degree again, and, of course, avoid having further illness. I planned to continue with my painting and my reading and, having just completed reading a very enjoyable book on Australia by Bill Bryson, entitled *Down Under*, was embarking on another by the same author on Shakespeare. At this time too I was writing about my experiences and hoped to complete this in July and, although I was not yet sure about how to do this, publish it in book form. My next door neighbour, Jack Rorke, himself an author of two books, encouraged me and gave me useful information on how to publish, including how to register and obtain an ISBN code number. What he was unable to advise on was how to get a suitable publisher.

Almost exactly seven months to the day from my stroke, Moira and I went to see Professor Dennis at his outpatient clinic in the Western General Hospital for a final check, as well as to discuss medication. We were glad we used the taxi service since car parking and restrictive barriers would have made things extremely difficult. We witnessed some of the frustration and difficulties other patients had. The Professor seemed pleased to see me, and though he said little and did not examine me, it was decided that from his point of view correct early decisions had been made and no change in medication should be effected. The reasons for this were discussed fully and honestly, and I was in agreement. Strangely, after this visit I for the first time felt a little sad; perhaps it was because the day was cold and foggy; perhaps I had expected the Professor to say how well I was doing, or at least give me some indication that all was well; but at least I was discharged with no need to see him again. My spirits were raised again when coincidentally an editorial in the *British Medical Journal* on strokes was published. It confirmed that I had been very lucky in having received stroke care as an inpatient in a stroke centre, as well as planned home care packages. Studies have shown the functional status of a stroke person at six months is associated with long-term survival, which is independent on age and stroke subtype. Stroke units have been shown to improve independence and survival at six months, as can early supported discharge by a specialised stroke team – which I consider I have had.

The next day I felt better and the weather was slightly less foggy. Daylight was beginning at about 7 a.m. and lasted until 5.30 p.m., which would give me more scope for my walking trips. I awoke to the sounds of aircraft at the airport revving up and taking off in the distance and the gradually increasing murmur of the cars in the main road as people went to work. At least I no longer was one of these! It was too early in the season to have the dawn chorus, but I heard a few sounds – notably the distant song thrush, the ever present trilling hedge sparrow, and the squealing of a flock of seagulls, presumably visiting a nearby rubbish dump or landfill site. My walk outside in late morning was the longest to date and lasted about forty-five minutes, even though it was quite cold and windy. I was very pleased at my stamina as well as the distances I now seemed to be able to go, which allowed me to visit areas further from my home. During this I heard few birds singing – probably because of the colder temperature – but noted a few crocuses and daffodils were present in sheltered spots in a few gardens. The afternoon involved a visit to see Julie for physiotherapy at McLeod Street, and again this helped to raise my spirits, for she reported that she could see a definite improvement in my shoulder movements. I was given some small objects to take home to practise hand and finger exercises, which I must admit I had not been doing recently.

The question of mild weather was of considerable interest to someone like me as it was helpful in both mood and the possibility of getting out. An interesting newspaper article on this very subject that same day discussed the fact that in the last two decades the mean February temperatures in Edinburgh has been climbing with a steady figure of about 5°C for the past five years, with a peak of 8° in 1998. Last January was the wettest in Edinburgh for more than one hundred years and gave nearly three times the average amount of rainfall. Joanna Vallely, the author, argued that global warming, if it exists, and the long term effects on flora and fauna have to be watched for and may not always be good ones.

I found that during February I had more time to listen to and read about news, and apart from the continuing saga on the weather changes throughout the world, not just in Britain, there were interesting debates on DNA population data collection for use in crime detection versus public concern about confidentiality, the high costs of gas and oil, pensions, biofuels, 'carbon footprints', immigrants, the Scottish scene in football and rugby, and of course, the continuing public concerns with wars and disasters abroad. The TV at home provided an almost continuous coverage for news as well as sport, given the greater variety of programmes available to me by satellite. Apart from these, I found the most interesting programme to be the wildlife one called *Life in Cold Blood* by Sir David Attenborough shown on BBC1. In this, unique pictures of frogs, lizards, chameleons and snakes abounded and enthralled – but of course I have always loved wildlife! The most relaxing programmes were usually golf tournaments, and the most irritating were the many cooking, celebrity renditions and property makeovers!

In our house, the most interesting change related to a conversion of our bathroom, which involved changing our bath, toilet, and sink. The work was completed efficiently within five days and made showering and bathing much easier for me, especially as I was now able to walk in myself and did not have to be lowered into the bath by means of a special chair arrangement. (It was much easier for Moira also.) Thanks to David, Bobby, and their excellent team of joiners, plasterers, electricians and plumbers, who made what could have been a messy and exhausting time a relatively pleasant experience – though admittedly the dry spell of warm weather also helped in that some of the preparative work could be done outside.

The weather towards the end of February was gusty, and walking for me outside was much more precarious, especially with the poor state of the local pavements. During this time I was able to finish reading Bryson's book on Shakespeare and in the process learned how little is actually known about his life. There may even be doubt as to who did write some of his work. I learned too that he created many words and phrases in use today, such as: antipathy, barefaced, leapfrog, zany, and 'one fell swoop', 'the milk of human kindness', 'be cruel to be kind' etc. Certainly, had I not been in my less active situation because of my stroke, I would probably not have read the book. A further interesting read was *Rolf on Art*, in which he discussed famous painters such as Monet, Van Gogh, Degas and Gauguin, and the sculptor, Rodin. A man of considerable abilities himself, Rolf Harris was able to attempt to recreate some of their paintings in their style and in some instances may have done better! Again, this was a book that I enjoyed more because of my newly found interest in painting. One of my walking indoor visits to the Gyle Shopping Centre resulted in the purchase of a very useful book, *The Writers' Handbook 2008*, in which I hoped to learn more about writing a book and how to approach a publisher. Out of a surprisingly large number there seemed to be about twenty that might be worthwhile approaching by writing to them or through their websites.

During the last week of the month I was still fortunate to be attending the physiotherapy under the care of Julie, and after each visit I felt extremely happy with her advice and with the new exercises she gave me. Even though my progress with regard to my hand and arm seemed slow, she was quite certain I was making progress. She made a suggestion regarding walking and going up and down stairs based on my improved walking strength, which meant I could walk with a greater stride action and climb stairs in a more natural and rapid action instead of the slower method, whereby I had to go up step by step with both feet on the same step before moving to the next one. I was able to try both of these when I got home and I think the walking action was more efficient and much less tiring, as was climbing the stairs. She also suggested that I could link up with another of her stroke patients, who was attending a gym and also went swimming in a nearby sports centre, to build up my strength. He apparently was happy to show me the ropes, and in fact I had met him on one of my previous visits to the McLeod Street Clinic. Lenny was his name, and armed with his telephone number and the fact that he appeared to have had an almost identical stroke as mine (but was further on with his recovery), it seemed to be a good idea to be in touch at some future date. A call was made that evening and he seemed keen to help me, so we arranged a meeting at the sports club during March. It was also of interest to me that Lenny was also using the same hand splint as me and was able to drive a modified motor car to get himself about.

The coming weekend not only heralded in March, but was also going to be my first away from home; the first visit to Aberdeenshire since my stroke, and also the first night staying in a hotel – quite a daunting prospect, but one that I felt I was ready for! Added to that apprehension was the fact that the day and night before were very windy and wet, and Moira would be the sole car driver. However, as it transpired, the weather conditions for travelling both to and back during the weekend were dry and sunny. It was marvellous to feel the freedom of being able to see the countryside again and to be able to travel away from home, even though it was a journey I had often made in the past.

The first difference I noted was the fact that there were no tolls to pay at the Forth Road Bridge – this had been abolished a few weeks previously! As a passenger, I found I had more time to look at the scenery than before, and probably now viewed it with keener interest! Most of the fields were either being ploughed, had been ploughed, or were showing signs of early green crop growth; some of the others had numerous molehills. The distant hills had an icing of snow and the deciduous shrubs and trees provided an interesting skeletal pattern in the foreground as well as the background. In some, where the new buds were beginning, there was a hint of a green haze. Apart from that the only splash of colour was provided by the yellow flowering gorse bushes in some fields and by the roadside and the many plantations of green conifers. On the outskirts of Edinburgh and Dundee, and to a lesser extent, Aberdeen, it was disappointing to see many plastic bags or parts of these stuck to bushes and trees, spoiling the appearance of the roadsides – very topical in view of the current debate in the media on the need to consider the use of plastic bags and our environment and the effect on wildlife! It was good to see some yellow-clad official individuals picking up some of this at the roadside about twenty-five miles from Edinburgh. The most frequent living things I saw were large flocks of rooks either foraging in the fields or swirling about on high, presumably getting ready to breed. Our route was fairly clear of roadworks except on the outskirts of Aberdeen, and we were held up a bit. We made better progress once through and reached our destination in Inverurie, the Strathburn Hotel, where we were to spend a very pleasant and comfortable stay overnight.

The main purpose of our visit, apart from seeing how I would manage, was to see our Aberdeenshire relatives, notably Moira's mother, who now lived in Inverurie, as did Sheila and Norman, my sister-in-law and brother-in-law. We met them for a most enjoyable evening meal in our hotel along with our other Aberdeen relatives, Moira's other sister, Edna, and husband Ron.

We returned to Edinburgh on the following day, which being a Sunday, was easier because of less traffic and no delays with roadworks, and I definitely felt that a further positive step had been undertaken with regard to my return to a more normal life. Moira agreed and I think also enjoyed her trip, apart from the driving!

The next few days were very gusty and the cold wind did not make walking easy but I still managed at least thirty minutes each day round our local streets. I visited the GP, Dr Donald, for a check-up – this was the monthly visit. My blood pressure was measured and apart from the systolic (upper) reading, was found to be satisfactory and still consistent with what was considered appropriate for me. However, I needed to take some more drugs!

I was on antibiotics for one week and a gastric acid reducing drug as well, because of a diagnostic endoscopy/dilatation examination I had during February for a long-term periodic swallowing difficulty had shown a small non-malignant narrowing at the lower end of my oesophagus and an organism called Helicobacter pylori in my stomach. Fortunately, I was now an expert tablet swallower, and the extra medication was not to be too much of a problem, and I did not seem to have any side effects. The new tablets were only to be taken for one week.

Neither the medication, the new dietary restrictions, nor my stroke appeared to have altered either my sleep pattern or the content of any dreams I could recall. The dreams were usually related to meetings, journeys, and friends; usually I had problems finding my car or keeping to a timetable, including also catching the train or plane to get away. Interestingly, in none was the stroke or any related problem even a part of it. Operations and the results featured on rare occasions, as did clinical meetings and sport – usually golf.

Moira was feeling a lot more confident with me and she was able to go to a monthly outing with 'The Rosebuds' in town for a coffee morning that she thoroughly enjoyed. These meetings are usually held during the first week of each month and are for former nurses who had worked in the Western Infirmary in Glasgow in the past and now lived in or around Edinburgh. It was in this hospital that Moira and I met initially when she was a staff nurse and I was a resident house officer. I was now quite capable of being of being left to fend by myself for the mornings or the afternoons, and this gave me and Moira more independence and confidence.

However, it was during the second weekend of March that I began to feel a little sad and Moira began to show evidence of strain. Possibly this was partly the result of being on extra medication, and partly the result of her having the extra responsibility of looking after my aviary birds, which were extremely messy and took a lot of her valuable time, as did a tropical fish tank! In order to improve this I will have to consider these problems and arrive at a difficult, yet inevitable and sensible decision that will assist Moira. She has been extremely tolerant and helpful in my various hobbies over many years, and now that I require more personal care and am much less mobile I can no longer manage these things myself. I think at the very least that the tank and the few fish may have to be disposed of, though how to do this remains a problem and worry to me. With these difficulties it is probably not surprising that I felt down in the dumps. The apparent slow progress with regard to my hand and right shoulder probably also depressed me, though I appreciate that this was bound to take longer than my walking, which continues to come on splendidly. During the previous week I have been able to walk for thirty minutes on two occasions on the same day, and seem to be getting fitter and more confident. Overall, I consider that my spirit and optimism remain generally good. It is probably the case that at some times post-stroke episodes of reflection and depression are to be expected.

On 11 March I felt a bit better as I walked the greatest distance so far from my home to the junction with the Barnton Hotel (empty, for sale at present, and in a deteriorating condition) and back home in a time of forty-five minutes. Apart from some discomfort in my right shoulder, I felt very strong and invigorated and was able to withstand a stiff but intermittent wind – much kinder than other parts of the UK, where there was much destruction and damage associated with flooding as a result of a major storm coming across the Atlantic from North America and a high spring tide.

On this day as well, Moira and I went a short distance in our car to have a look at the local Leisure Centre at Drumbrae, which Julie Hooper, physiotherapist at the McLeod Street Clinic, had recommended for continuing my physiotherapy exercises. We met Lenny and his wife and were shown round the swimming pool and gymnasium and were impressed. It seemed that the costs of using these excellent facilities were very reasonable and it would be something that would benefit me. Certainly this was Lenny's view and he had been a keen 'user' for over one year! As I was going to see Julie the following day, I proposed to discuss with her what she would advise me to take part in. Lenny and his wife were keen to advise and help and, since he had suffered a similar stroke to mine almost two years ago, I felt his experience as well as his friendship would be of considerable value to me, as the future proved.

The visit to Julie was most useful again, and she gave me further exercises to strengthen my shoulder and arm. This included using a static pedal bike, an arm lifting device, and latex ribbons tied onto wall bars that I had to pull in various directions. The latter I would be able to replicate on our stairs at home while the others would be done under supervision at the Leisure Centre, and for this she was going to send a referral form. There would also be some benefit in the swimming pool, as water does give increased support to the body, especially useful for my arm and hand but a little less convenient for me and Moira, who would have to dry and change me after this in order to save time and for safety. I still could not put on socks and shoes on without help.

A letter arrived from a representative of the NHS inviting me to complain, if I wished, regarding the observations which I had given to Jackie Sansford on the day of my discharge from the Victoria Hospital. After careful consideration, I decided that as I had received from her a promise that she would look into them, I did not need to formally complain any further. The main issue as far as I was concerned was the shortage of therapists, especially when the unit claimed to be a rehabilitation centre. I think this is a universal problem that is related to money allocation and is not due to lack of trained persons. Whether anything would develop from this was probably doubtful, whatever I did or said!

The main things that were due to happen over the last two weeks of March would be a review visit to the urology clinic, a visit to the gym, and a visit for several days from Alan, Susanna, and our grandson Joshua prior to their holiday in Austria. I was looking forward to the latter visit but not the former! A telephone call from Jennie, one of the hospital volunteers on 19 March cheered me up greatly. I learned that £3,000 had been donated to the unit, possibly in part as a result of my short report at the Cruden's lunch in December. It was agreed that I would visit the volunteers and the unit on 31 March, and at this time I could show some of the newer paintings that I had done at home including one of 'Daisy' – a beloved rag doll belonging to one of our neighbours, Ann, which apparently accompanied her wherever she went, even on holiday and on visits to her dentist and doctor! This, I hoped, might be suitable to make into a gift or even a Christmas card. I would also be able to give the volunteers a copy of my illustrated article to be published in *Surgeons' News* on left-handedness ('Turn to the left').

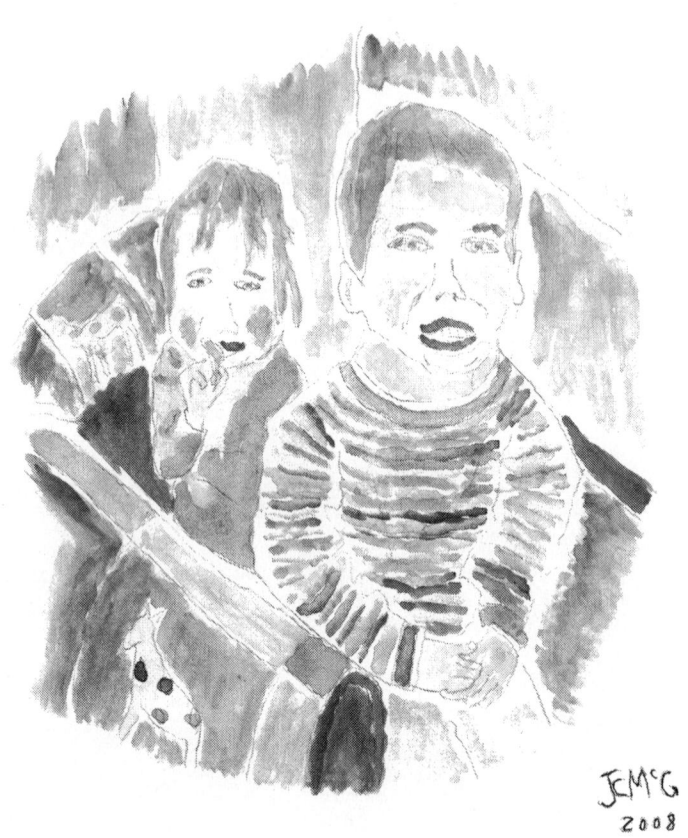

JcMcG
2008

HOLLY and CALLUM

Spring – It's Official!

Easter was earlier than usual this year, and in fact the last time it was so early was in 1913. Thursday, 20 March was actually the spring equinox – equal day and night-time – as well as the official start of spring. The weather forecast for the start of the Easter weekend holiday period was not good, and it was predicted that it would be very cold and there could be snow! I had in fact already noticed that daylight in the mornings started earlier at about 6 a.m. and darkness fell at about 7 p.m. During my daily walks around the local area I saw more flowers such as crocuses, daffodils, and primulas. I also heard the tentative beginnings of blackbird songs, and saw sparring over territories by robins and blackbirds.

On the day in question the weather, though coldish, was certainly sunny and eminently suitable for my walk in the late afternoon. Earlier, I had visited the urology clinic in the Western General, and it was found that I was 'doing well' and, while I had to continue with the medication, I did not require surgery and would not need to be reviewed until September. This was a great relief to me and Moira! In the morning, Callum, our grandson, had been left with us. He behaved well, and gave me great enjoyment with his antics. In actual fact, seeing my grandchildren has given me considerable pleasure as well as giving me a real purpose to continue the quest for improvement in my recovery. I completed a painting of Holly and Callum and was reasonably pleased with the result. I find doing faces quite difficult to fashion in a realistic way, apart from trying to get the correct colouring – a bit ironic for a former plastic and cosmetic surgeon!

Easter Friday, or Good Friday, was initially cold but sunny, with a few scattered snow showers in the evening but the snow did not lie. In the afternoon I visited the Leisure Centre to receive my initial assessment for my rehabilitation for gym work. For this I was seen and looked after by Ayla, who was a lovely twenty-one-year-old girl who seemed young enough to be a daughter or even a granddaughter of mine! Various questions were asked about my medical history and my personal aims. Then my blood pressure and weight were measured, but the apparatus for measurement of my body fat indicated an 'error' and thus remains a mystery! I was given a trial on a rowing apparatus and a static cycle, and showed that I could use these in future, but was advised to purchase sport trainers for future visits. At the next visit I would be shown some weight apparatus and possibly the walking treadmill, and an appointment for the following week was made as I left. Subsequently, Moira took me to a sports shop in the Gyle Centre, where a suitable, comfortable pair of the required shoes was purchased, and coincidentally I was able to put in useful walking practice with them that evening.

Easter Sunday morning was dry, sunny, windless and cold. I walked for thirty minutes in my new trainers round our estate without problem and, apart from the plaintive piping notes of great tits, the occasional outburst of hedge sparrows' little songs, and the raucous cawing of common crows, I saw and heard little evidence of bird life. More colour was to be seen in the gardens, and cherry blossom, together the occasional camellia and flowering redcurrant, adding an attractive pink to the yellow daffodils and variegated primulas.

Today we are expecting the arrival of Alan, Susanna, and Joshua from Delhi, and received an early morning telephone call from Alan that they had arrived in London Heathrow. However, the flight to Edinburgh had been delayed – the last thing one would wish after a long flight from India! To add to their discomfort, only one of their two cases had arrived in Edinburgh and they had to wait at Heathrow most of the day before they got a flight to Edinburgh and eventually to our home.

I have started to read another book – one which I had meant to read before my illness but didn't seem to have the time then! This was a book on Leonardo da Vinci, who was one of my heroes from the past, and written by Michael White. One of the first things I learned about him was that he was a left-handed, illegitimate, vegetarian homosexual who received no formal education but whose career as a painter, scientist, musician, and inventor took off when he left home and received training in Florence and then went to Milan. He recorded much of his work, including anatomical dissections, as truly exquisite and accurate drawings. This book promised to be most interesting, if perhaps rather a 'heavy read'. Time will tell whether I will be able to complete it, but time now should not be a factor at least.

Good news today on Easter Monday – the lost suitcase was delivered by the airport courier service at lunchtime!

All of our visitors had a good night's sleep, and our young grandson, Joshua, proved to be full of smiles and action as he crawled about our floors and played with some musical toys. A visit from Edna, Ron, and my nephew (their son) Richard, before lunch, gave us real pleasure and a chance for all to exchange news and an update of our family affairs.

Contrary to the reports of wintry weather in other parts of the country, the good bright weather seemed to be a feature in Edinburgh, and this encouraged me to go in the afternoon for what would be to date my longest walk, lasting about one hour round the complete circuit of our area – something that I had never even done before my stroke! I did not feel too tired after this, but reckoned I might find tomorrow's visit to the gym 'interesting' to say the least!

The visit to the gym went fine and I managed to do longer on the cycle and rowing machine, though it was clear that my stamina was still an issue. A new element designed to try to improve my upper body and shoulder strength was introduced. This involved the use of a medicine ball and some light weights which I found, as expected, to be quite difficult. Later that day I drew and painted a picture of Joshua to complete the grand-children's series! I think I have managed to capture his face and look realistically.

It was Alan's birthday today, 26 March, and to celebrate this we went out for an evening meal at Lauriston Farm with Susanna, Joshua, Trudy and Holly. Andrew was in New York on business, while Callum was in Arbroath with his other grandparents. It was a very enjoyable meal and night out for me and the others.

The main thing in the newspapers at this time, apart from the usual celebrity scandals, that was interesting to me was a debate about the use of animal-human embryos eventually for use in treating certain otherwise untreatable diseases, and the opposition from various persons, religious groups and others. A further interesting feature was the publication of a garden bird watch study from the RSPB for 2008, which was carried out over a weekend in January by nearly 27,000 Scottish people. This was something in which I had taken part in previous years, but owing to my recovering condition I had not done so this year. The current results showed the chaffinch to be the most commonly sighted, but the blackbird was the most widely seen species, in about 92% of gardens. The siskin (a finch) appeared for the first time in the top ten at number 10, possibly because of colder temperatures in Europe and milder winters in Scotland. It's not a bird that I have noticed in my area, but this will give me something to look out for.

Though more spring flowers were now in evidence I have not seen any butterflies or honeybees as yet, though a single bumble-bee has flown and been seen by me in our front garden on several days recently. As there is currently considerable worry amongst the honeybee keepers about a lethal parasite killing bees, it will be interesting to study this during my walks in the warmer months. It is lucky that I have always had a great interest in natural history, as it will give me an extra feature to aid my recovery.

On Saturday, 29 March, Moira and I were up earlier than normal in order to see Alan, Susanna, and Joshua away on their trip to ski in Austria. Moira took them to Edinburgh Airport in our car. We greatly enjoyed their visit to see us and we hoped they also had had an enjoyable stay. We look forward to seeing them again in June, when they plan to stay longer in Scotland, and Alan will be looking for a new career, as well as a home. I will find this to be an interesting event to look forward to.

Daylight was now starting at about 5 a.m. and going on until about 7.15 p.m. and, while the dawn chorus was limited to a single blackbird and the hedge sparrows, this was probably to be expected at this early part of the year. Summer time was due to start tomorrow, so we would have to remember to move the clocks one hour forward!

I managed to complete the reading of the book on Leonardo

da Vinci although I have to admit that I found it pretty heavy to read and I tended to 'scan read' towards the end. For anyone interested in studying the history and contribution of Leonardo to the Renaissance, his art, his anatomical dissections and accompanying drawing records, his optical and bird flight studies, his designs for harnessing water, his designs for war machinery and musical instruments etc, this book is for them. In many ways he was an amazing man both talented and gifted in many ways as well as being well ahead of many discoveries to be 'made' by others in later centuries! The main feature of his life was his artistic ability particularly in a three-dimensional way, his obsession with an enquiring mind and observation, and his written record keeping – not bad, given his poor start in life and lack of basic education.

On the last day of March I paid a visit to ward 9 at the Royal Victoria Hospital and saw some of the volunteers and nurses. I was well received, of course, and was able to relate how I was progressing. The patients were mostly new to me, suggesting that the turnover was good. I recognised one youngish man who had been in when I had first been admitted and spoke with Jacki, a woman who came into the unit about one month after me and, though improving, still had no idea as to how much longer she would be an inpatient for. She hoped to be able to go to see her daughter in Vancouver in August of this year and possibly stay and work in that city. She admitted that she had been periodically subject to being depressed because of her illness and situation, but was at present feeling better, and was pleased to see how well I was doing as it raised her spirits. She too had plans to write about her experience as a patient, with a view of presenting an optimistic account that could help other patients.

I was able to give the volunteers a copy of my article due to be published on left-handedness, as well as my painting of 'Daisy', which I hoped they could make up some gift cards. A recent painting I had made of a long-tailed tit was also selected for the same purpose by the volunteers, and they confirmed they would be interested in looking at possible paintings for next Christmas some time in the future.

In the afternoon Moira took me for my next gym appointment

and I went on the bicycle and rowing machine for slightly longer than the last time, though I still find my fitness is not too good as yet; but then I never before my illness went to any such places!

I also started reading another book. This time I hope it will not be such a heavy read, but will be equally as interesting and revealing on evolution and in particular the mind of Charles Darwin in the Galapagos Islands.

April promises to be a very interesting month, and I hope to progress further with the fitness aspect as well as making some progress in improving my right shoulder function; though I feel I am realistic with regard to slower and unpredictable recovery there compared with my leg.

April – a Month of Activity

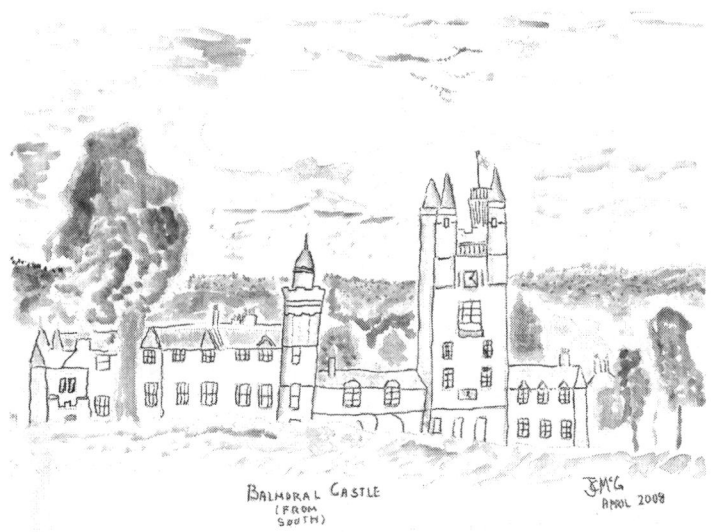

BALMORAL CASTLE
(FROM
SOUTH)

JMcG
APRIL 2008

April the first is sometimes called April Fool's Day and, though I often tried to catch out Moira, I had no suitable ideas this year, and she was looking out for some jape anyway! I did however successfully recognise a highly imaginative and impressive hoax on the BBC TV breakfast show – flying penguins in Antarctica! This had been presented as a new wildlife scoop but was admitted the following morning on the same programme to be a computer-ised animation. This was in contrast with the wonderful wildlife production currently underway by the wildlife BBC team in India using elephants who carried remotely controlled cameras to produce unique and intimate pictures of tigers and other rarely seen creatures (*Tiger – Spy in the Jungle*).

During the same morning Moira and I made a startling, but in retrospect simple, discovery that explained why my recent outside walks had been more difficult – a new battery for my foot-heel control box! We do not remember being advised on this when it was fitted – perhaps it should have been obvious! A telephone discussion with Lenny, who also had a similar apparatus, was able to clarify what to do; he also made the sensible suggestion that we should take an extra battery with us when we were away from home.

The following day was not one that I was looking forward to as I was due to visit the dentist and get a tooth out. It was a nice sunny morning, however and a half-hour walk around our area and a hot chocolate break mid-morning seated in our back garden helped to keep spirits up. I am very fortunate in that the back garden area is quite large, has been carefully and professionally landscaped by Mr J Northam, our long-time gardener, and abuts a small oak wood. When the weather warms up, I will be able to sit out and enjoy the scene, read and perhaps paint. During my brief stay outside I noted a queen wasp and a bumblebee as well as a peacock butterfly flying about, and heard wrens, hedge sparrows, greenfinches, and a wood pigeon singing forth. The visit to the dentist was surprisingly non-traumatic and the tooth in question – a wisdom one – was extracted quickly and efficiently by the lady dentist under local anaesthetic.

During the next night I slept reasonably well without the need to take any analgesics. I had been advised not to take non-prescribed aspirin as this might cause extra bleeding, but could continue my usual prescribed medication, which included a daily dose of aspirin. I did dream, and can remember that it involved sitting a clinical examination with a patient and sitting down for a meal with others afterwards! I awoke at about 5 a.m. when it was still dark and for the next hour heard the dawn chorus, which consisted of large numbers of blackbirds warbling from various parts around our house – not the fluid song that probably comes later on in the warmer weather. This outburst seemed to stop suddenly after one hour, leaving almost complete silence apart from the sounds of early traffic on the main road and aircraft at the airport.

Kay, one of the hospital volunteers, brought samples of cards with my painting of 'Daisy' in the afternoon, and seemed pleased at the end result. The day before another volunteer, Jenny, had brought a card she had made from my painting of the long-tailed tit, which she was also pleased with – and so was I! Both of these cards were considered worthy of being suitable for using for selling for unit funds for the Stroke Service. I also hoped I would be able to use them in this book.

The coming weekend promised to be interesting as well as exciting, as Moira and I were due to go to have a short break with the 'Rugby Crowd' at a hotel in Ballater.

The trip away was planned carefully several months ago in conjunction with the 'Rugby Crowd' as part of our long-standing yearly weekend away break. As mentioned before, this group of friends had been of great support to me and Moira over the years and throughout my hospitalisation. All of them except Jacqui, who had to attend a family event, were planning to go, and this would be a further step for my rehabilitation. It had been agreed that we should go to Ballater, and a suitable hotel was selected. The weather forecast for the weekend had been predicted to be very cold and snowfalls were thought to be likely in most of Britain, but especially in the north of Scotland.

Moira and I left on the Friday morning just after 10 a.m. and made our way north. It was a very pleasant drive in dry and sunny conditions, which made the views on the journey a real advert for the beautiful scenery of Glenshee, the Cairngorms, and the forests and moors around Balmoral, Braemar, and Ballater. The stunning views of the high Cairngorm Mountains, some topped with a covering of sparkling white snow, and the wide bubbling River Dee, gave me a great lift. At one magical point on the hillside near the road we saw a small herd of red deer moving slowly and close enough to make out the majestic stag's antlers.

The hotel we stayed in for the next two nights – the Glen Lui – was comfortable, probably just suitable for a disability such as mine, run by a family, and had an excellent menu for breakfast and evening meals. The bedrooms were small and unfortunately the shower facility in our room was quite unsuitable and unsafe for me to use. I understand improvements are underway and the current owners, who have only recently taken on the hotel, are keen to improve and upgrade the facilities. It would not at present be possible as far as I could see for a wheelchair-bound person to have access to any bedroom in the main hotel, as there is no lift but there were outside ground level lodges available for use.

Saturday was going to be our main day of activity and we were lucky in having Ros Newlands with us as one of the 'Rugby Crowd'. She was our 'team organiser', and coincidentally is the current President of the World Federation of Tourist Guides Association, as well as a member of the Scottish Tourist Guide Association in which she is Training Manager and Course Director. She was able to plan and advise us on where we might go and visit, and has been of great assistance on the previous trips we have made over many years. After a general discussion it was decided we should go to Balmoral and possibly try a 4 x 4 safari around the estate that was advertised as one of the attractions. Unfortunately this was not available on our weekend, but we decided to go to Balmoral in any case and explore.

Balmoral has been the highland retreat of the Royal Family since 1852, and is probably well known throughout the civilised world. Provided they are not in residence, it is usually open for visitors to explore the grounds, see any exhibitions, have meals in the refectory, buy items in a shop, and visit the ballroom. The accessibility for those like me or wheelchair-bound individuals is, as to be expected, very good. While there are disabled parking facilities in the outside car park, it is possible, as we did, to use our disabled sticker, and be allowed to go in and park near to the main castle, thus saving a not inconsiderable walk or wait for a tractor-driven carriage. If I had wanted one, motorised wheelchairs were also available for hire. I had been there on at least one occasion several years before, but this time was special, and perhaps I was going to be more observant! The first thing to notice was the great quietness and the clear air of the locality, apart from the beautiful castle and surrounding grounds/estate. No wonder the Queen and her family enjoy the area so much!

A quote from Queen Victoria, whose remarks, found in the guidebook on Balmoral which I purchased, seem apt:

It was so calm and so solitary it did one good as one gazed around; and the pure mountain air was most refreshing. All seemed to breathe freedom and peace, and to make one forget the world and its sad turmoils –

While all of our crowd did their own thing, including walking out into the grounds, Moira and I explored the perimeter of the castle, the ballroom, the exhibitions of art, gowns, carriages, the shop and the tearoom. This gave me a good walk and much enjoyment, even though by this time the weather was changing, with periodic squally snow flurries.

After a lunch break in the tearoom, our group decided to explore the surrounding areas in our cars and possibly visit Glen Muick and a visitor centre there. Those who wished would be able to go for a longer walk in the area, weather permitting of course. Getting to the Glen Muick area proved slightly more difficult than expected because of one road being closed to the public, but it gave us a long distance view of Birkhall, which is a secluded holiday retreat of some members of the Royal Family. Someone of importance must have been there, as one of the entrance roads was guarded by a Metropolitan Policeman! The car journey gave me a great opportunity to study the trees, the mountains and the moorlands, in between what were becoming increasingly frequent snowfalls and surprisingly sunny periods.

Looking at the colours of the trees and the moors was extremely interesting and revealing of the beautiful variations of greens, greys, whites and purples. The trees were not all evergreen pines and there were a large number of silver birches, both lining the roads and in the middle distance; many of them guarded the road verges like vast armies of straight, white-barked soldiers. Those further back were older and larger but all had a purple bloom haze-like effect caused by their emerging buds, which contrasted with the evergreen pines and a lighter green from trees such as larches, also beginning to bud forth. Some of the tree barks were covered by greyish-green lichens – a sure sign of a healthy atmosphere – which added to the colour patterns provided by the green mosses that covered the forest floor.

Suddenly, the trees gave way to stark moorlands and vistas of rolling hills and mountains covered near their summits with snow, and below with scattered grey boulders and a purple mass of heather, even though the flowers were still to come out. We were fortunate in seeing a large group of red deer; something had caused them to seek lower ground. Perhaps they knew something we were about to find out later in the day! We all arrived safely at the car park of the Loch Muick reserve, having travelled along narrow roads by a river on one side and the picturesque mountains on the other. A short walk downhill took us to a nature display in a small building that gave examples of the Cairngorm wildlife to be found and protected. The plans of some of us to walk farther afield were changed by what seemed to be the reason why the deer were seeking lower ground – namely worsening weather and snowfalls. Accordingly, we returned post haste to our hotel! This turned out to be a wise decision as the snow fell almost continuously all night and by the next morning it was lying about five centimetres deep.

The last evening in our hotel was none the less very enjoyable, and we had an excellent meal there. We had a small group sweepstake on the Grand National horse race which had been run earlier that afternoon. We each drew three or four horses and put in a small sum to cover. The winner of our sweepstake was Ros – the horse being 'Comply or Die', which was the joint favourite. Generously, she elected to donate this to a charity (the Kovalam project), which we contribute towards as a group following the tsunami disaster, which affected this village in India near Chennai in late December 2004.

The story surrounding this is quite interesting, in that it arose from our 'Rugby Crowd' group who came to Alan and Susanna's wedding held at Fisherman's Cove Hotel in March 2005; it is a few miles down the coast south of Chennai. The tsunami had destroyed fishing boats and dwellings. A meeting took place with a village representative who had lost a relative and was in touch with a British lady, Sylvia, who was an organiser of a charity for the village. As a result, each year our group collect some money for the village and this has gone towards rebuilding a school, the provision of educational material, and 'adoption' of two young brothers called Rashmutheen and Shalimetheen. This act, coordinated by Ros and Alf and Sylvia, has further cemented the unique association of our 'Rugby Crowd', which has existed since our sons left school in 1993 or thereabouts.

In the morning we awoke to find a considerable fall of snow had occurred and a real Christmas-like scene greeted us around the hotel. We debated how best to try to drive home. I felt very frustrated that I was unable to assist Moira, either with driving or luggage etc. It was decided that it would be safer to go home via Aberdeen rather than the shorter, but almost certainly snowier, route through Glenshee. This proved to be a wise and surprisingly easy road and, while initially we drove through snow and blizzard conditions, by the time we reached the outskirts of Aberdeen, and from then on to Edinburgh, we saw no snow. Moira and I arrived home in mid-afternoon to a sunny but cold Edinburgh, tired but happy with our weekend break. There was no doubt that the trip away from home had done us both good as well as boosting my confidence.

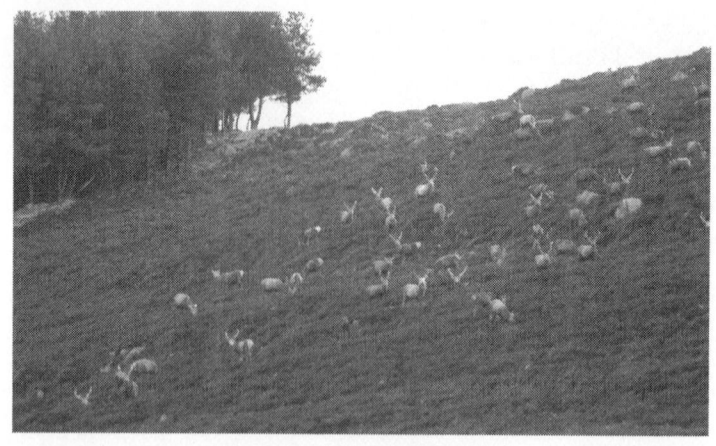

Deer at Glen Muick

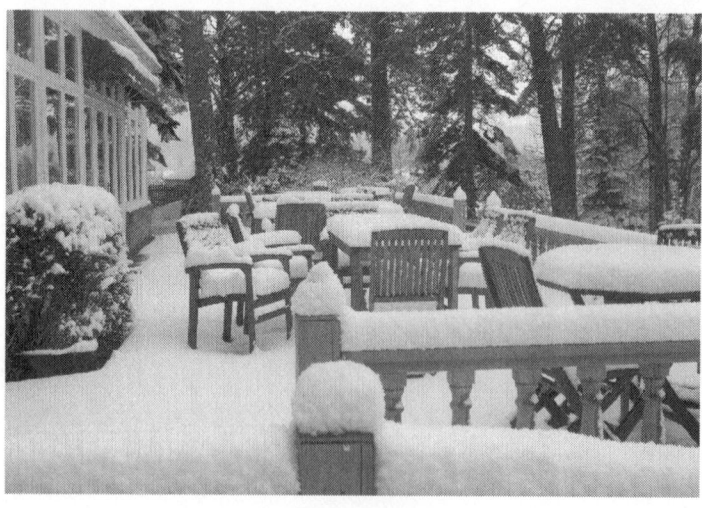

Snow at Ballater

Photographs courtesy of Mr Allan Smith

Continued Activity

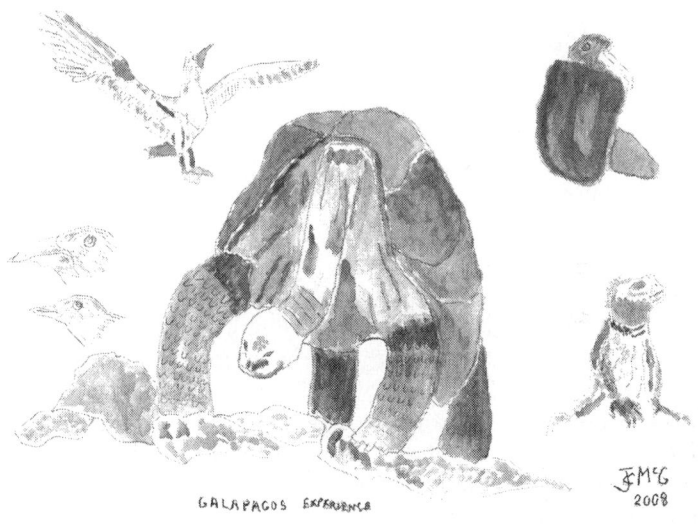

GALAPAGOS EXPERIENCE

JMcG
2008

Painting of Galapagos features

A further visit to see Ayla at the Drumbrae Leisure Centre gave me the chance of progression with exercises – I did ten minutes on the bike, which was double my previous effort, and further trunk exercises using a large beach ball. Additionally I spent a short time on a rowing machine and an apparatus designed to strengthen shoulder movement backwards and forwards. Ayla is very gentle but seems to be keen and well aware of my disability and my requirements. She had just been accepted for a new module for training specifically for strokes and expressed interest in meeting up with Julie Hooper, should this be possible. This was something that would likely be of considerable help to me in my recovery. As I was due to visit Julie the next day for physiotherapy, it seemed that this would be a chance to discuss this further.

Julie was keen to learn about Ayla and what exercises I had thus far being doing. She was happy with these and said she would be pleased to meet with Ayla and discuss her involvement with the new modules. She also felt that I had made good progress with my shoulder and gave me a new list of exercises to try. Appointments with her could now be extended to once per month, especially since I was attending Ayla once a week.

Jennie, one of the Victoria Hospital volunteers, telephoned to report that orders for my two recent cards – 'Daisy' and the long-tailed tit – which our 'Rugby Crowd' had made during our recent trip to Ballater, were going ahead. Apparently, these cards are currently on sale to hospital visitors for the funds at the cost of £1.50 each!

10 April was a day when I went to the diabetic clinic at the Western General, where I was reassured to learn my diabetes was well controlled and it would now be possible to reduce the metformin tablets from two twice daily to one twice daily. A further appointment was to be in August, around about which time I will have my eyes tested again to check that no diabetic or hypertensive effects have developed; none have so far. My blood pressure was measured, and in keeping with my GP's checks showed the systolic value still to be a little higher than normal, though the lower diastolic figure was normal. Whether the higher result should or could be lowered further and safely remains an outstanding problem that, I must confess, I do not fully have a view on, nor I believe do the doctors. Though this is somewhat worrying, I am quite prepared to remain optimistic, especially as I feel well and have no adverse symptoms.

The newspapers of the day were interesting from a number of things, medical as well as non-medical. Prince Charles and his wife Camilla had been in Ballater and, though it was not mentioned, they were possibly the reason for the policeman we saw at the entrance to Birkhall a few days before. A national poll by the *Scottish Daily Mail* 'showed a dramatic surge over recent months in the number of people backing a separate Scotland', and a report in the *Scotsman* by the Marine Conservation Society showed that 'a tide of plastic waste swamps Scotland's filthy beaches'. Obviously we need as a nation to try to 'clean up'; whether this threat to the Union is going to be or not to be remains at this day a decision yet to be decided upon.

With regard to medical matters, both papers had reports. The *Scotsman* had an interesting report on stem cell experiments that might eventually 'repair damage of strokes', though this was a few years in the future. The *Daily Mail*, in two separate medical reports, gave me some other interesting things to think about. The first article stated that taking regular exercise puts 'ageing on hold for twelve years' as well as tending to reduce stress levels. The second was a report that 'eating an egg a day increases the risk of premature death for middle-aged men, especially in diabetics'. Although I rarely eat eggs now, for many years I went to work on a boiled egg, and can remember the time when there was an advert advising us 'to go to work on an egg'! It all goes to show that all these medical advice stories should be taken with a pinch of salt, but in my case, of course, salt intake has to be restricted!

The television remains one of my main interests and this week, with major football matches, and the Major golf tournament in Augusta, promises to be a good one. Already I have watched Liverpool, Manchester United, Chelsea and Glasgow Rangers, who have succeeded in winning semi-final places in their respective European championships, and after the first round, the joint leader in the golf is British, and a number of other British golfers, including the Scot, Sandy Lyle, are amongst the leaders. I am fairly sure that sporting interest and success are good for the morale of spectators, myself, and the success of the working man in contributing to happiness of the nation.

I now intend to make a real bid to undertake the new shoulder exercises that Julie Hooper has given me to do at home, even though they are challenging and difficult. At least my walking continues to progress, and on one evening this week, I did my usual thirty-minute walk in our estate and was accompanied the whole way by Warwick, one of our neighbours, who kindly said he would like to walk with me. You might wonder why this was to me an accomplishment, but because of the need to walk and talk at the same time, this of course means more energy requirements and was thus a further step forward.

Trudy, unfortunately, has been admitted to the Royal Infirmary of Edinburgh with pneumonia, as a consequence of asthma and being pregnant. Fortunately she has not been affected too badly and was admitted as a precautionary measure. Moira and I were able to visit her in the evening and we saw that she was getting better. Hopefully she was going to get home within the next few days. (She did!)

On checking my pills for the ensuing week at the weekend on Saturday morning, it was noticed that I was 'short', and so a visit to the local chemist was required. Moira and I went there by car to sort this problem and this enabled me to walk back home – a distance of about half a mile or more. Though it was a cold and dull morning, there were a few birds singing – the usual tits, greenfinches, and hedge sparrows – but a song thrush and several melodious blackbirds performed in short bursts. I had heard a woodpecker tapping on tree trunks in local oak wood during the past week on one of my walks, but on this walk he chose to be silent... The gardens were becoming even more springlike, with copious daffodils, tulips, cherry blossoms, heathers, forsythia, and fragrant flowering redcurrants seen most commonly. All these giving a beautiful yellow and red backcloth to the evergreen trees and shrubs – the buds on others not quite opening out yet, though looking imminent and awaiting a warm day in the future week.

I received a card during the week from a Consultant Plastic Surgeon, Peter Mahaffey, who had been a junior colleague with me in Nottingham. Apart from wishing me well he commented that 'he was eternally grateful for all the encouragement and inspiration I had given him when he was starting out in Nottingham'. It's nice to be remembered in this way, as well as acting as a real tonic to my spirit!

On Sunday, 13 April, Moira and I went out for lunch with John Northam and Lydia at Gullane in the Golf Inn. The run in the car out from Edinburgh was one into East Lothian that I have always liked, with a nice mixture of farmland, coastal views of the Firth of Forth, and golf courses. The long plots of golden daffodils on the roadside on the way into Longniddrie are truly spectacular and by themselves made the journey worthwhile. Both the meal and the company were most enjoyable, and there was much talk about art and gardening. On the way home I observed the light green changes in the hawthorn bushes, sycamores and chestnut trees as leaves began to burst forth. As yet there was no sign of beech, oak or elm leaves. It was curious to note how the numerous silver birches lining the roadsides in places, although they had the ghostlike white bark, had many branches in their lower parts, giving a completely different appearance from the tidy regimented look of their brothers and sisters seen recently near Ballater. I wonder why this should be. Perhaps they are different races.

The weekend television was quite interesting, showing the London Marathon, which has a staggering number of participants. Apart from the elite athletes, there are many thousands of others, including wheelchair persons, taking part. Amongst those running for various charities were a man aged over one hundred years, a young lad who had been told as a child that he would never walk after a serious accident involving a head injury, a group of Masai warriors running and dancing to raise money for a water plant for their village, and many others – some dressed bizarrely and some doing unusual things as they went round the course, such as the lady on stilts and the person dressed as a robot and walking ever so slowly. Most of these and many others demonstrate great courage and determination.

Similarly, Queen of the South football team, also on the television, demonstrated great skill and determination in defeating Aberdeen – a team in the higher division – to reach the Final of the Scottish Cup. No doubt the whole of Dumfries will be excited for the next month or so, and the workforce will be encouraged and motivated! The golf at Augusta was as usual a wonderful television experience visually, in a venue embellished with azaleas, water and brilliant golfers, but spoiled a little from a British viewpoint in that no Brit featured in the top ten places, in spite of early promise. The champion, Trevor Immelman of South Africa, was a worthy winner who had led after each of the four rounds and apparently had had a serious operation last year, which made his victory more impressive and poignant.

I completed reading about the Galapagos Islands at the weekend. It was a most interesting account – the more so because Moira and I had been on a visit last year before my stroke. Perhaps I should have read the book beforehand and I would have appreciated even more the evolutionary significance of what have been described as 'the enchanted isles', and why Charles Darwin, after his visit in the nineteenth century, was stimulated to think and write about his own theories in *The Origin of Species*.

As far as my own evolution was concerned, I continued to work at Julie's shoulder exercises each day and found them fairly difficult as well as tiring. I also started each morning to get up and go down the stairs into the sitting room without using the foot stimulator, but still felt the need to use this for my walks outside. By now it was approaching the middle of what had been a busy period during April, and the second half promised to be equally so.

An Operation and the Rest of April

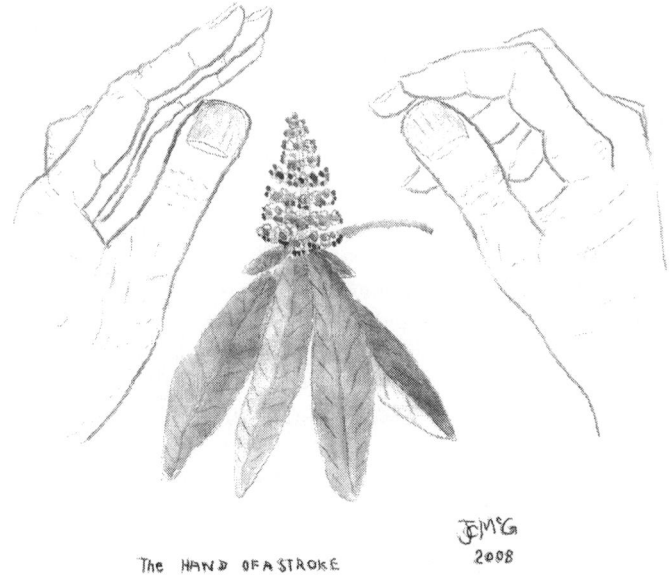

The HAND OF A STROKE

JEMcG
2008

Painting of chestnut blossoms and hands

The middle of April was upon us, and the 15th was a fine, sunny, warm day. The dawn chorus began at about 4.30 a.m. and finished at about 5 a.m. There was an eerie quietness over the ensuing two hours, presumably as the birds were looking for food or building nests. I had my usual walk early on in the morning and think I heard a chiffchaff calling in our oak wood. The walk was very pleasant and comfortable and it seemed even more springlike because the chaffinches were singing in greater numbers, their happy trills being as far as I am concerned one of the great sounds of spring.

Outside also, there are additional sounds and sights of men and machines working on our roads outside our house, as they repaired the road surface prior to insertion of 'sleeping policemen' as part of a more widespread project to slow down the traffic in our local roads. According to Tony, one of our neighbours, it took fifteen men and five hours to do this initial work, which resulted in resurfacing the road part in front of our house and left the rest of the road in our cul-de-sac untouched! It's a pity this does not apply to sorting our awful – and in places – dangerous pavements! In the course of my daily stroll I prefer to walk on the road where the pavements are worst. Fortunately, the stroke does not appear to have affected my balance, sight, or hearing and I am able to step out confidently from surface to surface and listen for oncoming traffic – in my view a most important thing for any ambulant stroke person. With regard to other senses such as smell and taste, these also seem unaffected, though I must admit the low fat and low salt foods have taken me some time to adjust to. The sense of smell has enabled me to enjoy the smell of lilies given by friends and relatives, the scent of flowering currants, newly cut grass, a creosoted fence, and in our front garden the less pleasant odour of a fox that had recently passed by and marked its territory.

Today, in the afternoon, I had my weekly visit to see Ayla and was introduced to some new exercises designed to strengthen my quads and hamstrings, in addition to the trunk and bike work. I increased my bike activity to two sessions of ten minutes without a problem, so my stamina had improved yet again. Just as well, as I had a further appointment later in the afternoon at Beechwood House – my previous consulting room site at Murrayfield Hospital – to see a former trainee, now a Consultant Plastic Surgeon, Stuart Hamilton. His job was to remove a small skin lesion under local anaesthetic from my left cheek. This he did with great skill and lack of discomfort. I was welcomed by the nurses, including Cecelia, one of the plastic surgery specialty nurses whom I worked closely with over many years, and who had been of great help in the management of my own patients. I would be returning to see her or her colleagues the following week for removal of the stitches.

It's almost nine months since my stroke, and I think I have made good progress in my recovery. I remain with a positive outlook and feel adjusted to my situation, though still frustrated at certain things such as not being able to use my right arm fully, not being able to drive a car, and not being able to play golf. However, these are things that could still be possible in due course and are worth aiming for. Every one who sees me has remarked how well I look, and physically I think this is a true picture, which has been helped by my normal facial appearance and relatively normal speech. Sometimes when I am tired or try to talk too quickly my words seem a little slurred, but my mental processes seem as sharp as ever!

A routine visit for an eye check-up was done during the week and reassuringly this showed no changes from my last visit one year ago, which was of course was before my stroke. In particular there were no diabetic or high blood pressure changes, but these will also be looked at by the diabetic clinic; next visit due in August.

There is no doubt that I feel less tired, and it was interesting that Moira found a fact sheet produced by the Chest, Heart and Stroke Scotland advice service, which contained useful information on strokes including a comment on 'fatigue' after strokes, indicating that it is common and lessens over time. A greater discussion paper was also found on the subject of fatigue that was first published in the Stroke Association's *Stroke News* in winter 2003. This study in Sweden suggested that slightly more women than men were affected, that it tended to occur in older patients who were in poorer general health before the stroke, and was more common when the right hemisphere was affected by a stroke. While it is recognised that the process of rehabilitation such as is required for walking, talking, eating, washing and physiotherapy requires 'colossal' effort, it is thought that the underlying causes are not fully explained by this. It is not related to stroke size and after two years it affects 10% of cases. There has been little research on treating post-stroke fatigue thus far. The use of antidepressants may not be helpful and may even worsen the fatigue, as may other medication taken. Unless it has been recognised by both patient and helpers it can 'slow recovery and even impair the ability to regain functions lost because of the stroke'. Exercise is advised to combat fatigue, but of course it should be realistic and supervised by the physiotherapists.

At this stage my laptop, which I had been using to type out this story, also gave in to serious fatigue, and when taken to our local 'mending shop' in Barnton, was pronounced irreparable. This was a blow, especially as I would lose several days of useful writing time as well as having to purchase a new laptop and having the worry of data transfer of all I had already written. I need not have worried about this – though I did! After seven days, including one day that was a public holiday, I was back to normal with a new laptop and my data intact, thanks to the excellent service from the DMC Computer Shop in Barnton – Gordon and John.

Quite a lot happened during the week concerned.

A visit to see the physiotherapists at Astley Ainslie Hospital to check on the ankle/foot stimulator occurred, and Katie and Jane were happy with how I was managing and how it was helping me. My stitches were successfully removed by the plastic surgery nurse, Cecelia, at Beechwood House, and I received a telephone call inviting me to come to be assessed for car driving because of a cancellation, which meant a much earlier appointment than I had believed would be the case. The date would be 21 April – not only the Queen's real birthday, but mine too! The referral for this assessment has and was made by the GP and was to the Scottish Driving Assessment Service, which is funded jointly by the NHS and the Transport Department of the Scottish Government. Referrals are also accepted from the DVLA, Motability, and solicitors. An in-car assessment can only be undertaken on people who have a current driving licence, but persons can be referred without one. I was warned that the assessment would take up to 2½ hours and would involve a physical assessment, a static unit assessment, and, as I had a driving licence, an in-car driving assessment. My appointment was to be at the Astley Ainslie Hospital Smart Unit in Edinburgh, but for those outwith Edinburgh a mobile service regularly visits hospitals in Aberdeen, Inverness, Dundee, Paisley, Irvine and Dumfries.

My appointment was for 9.15 a.m., which meant quite an

early start from home, but as Moira and I knew where to go we went by car and found easy and convenient parking outside a very modern Smart building. We were met by Sinead, an occupational therapist, whose job it was to see and examine me. I found the process extremely interesting, demanding and tiring. In the first place I had to read two number plates at a distance, and much to my surprise had some difficulty in reading one correctly – the one with numbers on a yellow background, and only two of the numbers concerned. The next task was done sitting at a table and involved copying coloured wooden shapes, matching road signs to road situations, and a memory test which consisted of delayed questions after I had a chance to read a paragraph on a road-related subject. All of these tests were fairly demanding, and though I did not get all correct I believe that I performed reasonably well. I doubt if I would have done any better before my stroke.

At any rate I was allowed to progress to the next stages, the first of which involved sitting in a static simulator and trying the brakes and accelerator in conjunction with reaction times initiated by a series of red lights. My reaction times were well within the normal, and it was ascertained that I would have to use my left foot to work the pedals as my right foot kept slipping off the pedals. In addition I was not capable of using my right hand to control the steering wheel, and so a special device would have to be fitted to the steering wheel for me to control turning and lights etc.

The final part of the test involved me driving in an adapted dual control car twice around the roads in Astley Ainslie Hospital – no mean feat, given that these roads are narrow and cars are parked at their sides! I felt I performed reasonably in view of the novelty of this experience. While Sinead gave little away, at least she did not indicate I would not be capable of driving eventually in a modified car and after a few lessons. A further visit in early May would be arranged to see if by wearing a foot splint (the one I had initially worn in the hospital before the stimulator) would make it possible for me to use my right foot for brake and accelerator pedals; this would mean fewer car modifications would be required. As Moira was keen for me to get a new chair to sit in, and there were possible ones exhibited in the same building for stroke people, we took the opportunity of staying after the car assessment and viewing these. One of these was chosen and arrangement was subsequently made for a home demonstration. As a result a few days later an order was made.

The following day I felt quite tired and took advantage of the sunny, warm day to sit outside in our garden and enjoy the sights and sounds. The first thing I noticed was the larger number of bumblebees touring around over the grass, presumably queens looking for possible nest sites or flowers to collect pollen from. As yet, I have not seen a single honeybee either in my garden or during my local walks outside. This apparent paucity of honey-bees has already been noticed nationwide and thought to be due to a mite-transmitted virus (varroa mite), or to an unknown cause which makes the bees fail to return to their hives (Colony Collapse Disorder). It is a very worrying matter and was even alluded to by Albert Einstein, who gave the following pro-nouncement: 'If the bee disappeared then man would only have four years of life left. No more bees, no more pollination, no more plants, no more animals, no more man.' Let's hope this will not come to pass!

The presence of a bird feeding station in the garden gave me an added interest for about 1½ hours. In particular, unlike the one in the Victoria Hospital grounds that I saw during my stay, ours had an anti-squirrel baffle which completely defeated these agile robbers. In fact, I have seen very few grey squirrels in our neighbourhood since I came home from hospital, and this seems to suggest a definite reduction from previous years; the cause for this is unknown. The most frequent visitors to the bird feeders were chaffinches followed by various tits and greenfinches with a ground-feeding pair of wood pigeons, a pair of stock doves, hedge sparrow, and robin on the area below the feeders where food debris fell down, dislodged by those feeding above. A surprising arrival of some starlings and a pair of jackdaws was noted at the feeders, acting like marauding pirates, while on a nearby tree a single magpie lurked but did not venture down.

The star turn, or turns, came towards the end of my sojourn when a pair of bullfinches came – the male sporting a bright red breast – and the real show-off, a greater spotted woodpecker that swooped down to the feeders. According to Moira, this bird always came to feed in the morning and at about 4 p.m. every day! Presumably, this was the same bird that had been tapping in the woods recently. Talking about tapping, the source of a curious light tapping sound which had puzzled me all afternoon was located to come from within a nest box on the side of one of our garden oak trees, and careful watching revealed the cause to be a nesting blue tit!

The next day Moira and I decided to visit the 2008 Mobility Roadshow, which had been advertised in the press and was only one of two that would be held in the UK this year. We made our way by car to the show, which was at the Royal Highland Centre, Ingleston, near Edinburgh and parked our car in the designated free car park beside the exhibition centre. Although we arrived near the advertised opening time we were amazed to find the car park was already full with thousands of visitors' cars. This confirmed the popularity of this meeting with the large numbers of people, many of whom were in wheelchairs. It made me feel very fortunate to be able to walk about the exhibition in relative ease, and also see the great variety of cars, motorised bikes, caravans, wheelchairs, and information booths offering advice on help for the disabled, including driving, holidays and parking permits. We learned that the *blue badge* used for disabled parking permit had to be accompanied by a clock when used in England, where only three hours' parking with it was allowed! Apart from the interesting visit, it was reassuring to see the amount of information and materials available for the disabled, as well as demonstrating to Moira and myself how much I was now able to walk about without discomfort. Thus at the end of April I was gaining in confidence in returning to the outside world; so much so that on the last Saturday in April I walked from my house non-stop to the entrance to the Burgess Golf Club and back, which was certainly the farthest distance yet I had achieved.

On the Sunday, Moira and I drove out for a lunch visit to a local garden centre in West Lothian. It was a lovely day with a temperature of about 13° Centigrade, and there was more evidence of trees coming into leaf – notably beech, sycamore, horse chestnut, rowan, birch, and willow, but not yet in oak or elm. The horse chestnut leaves with their droopy hand-like leaves provided a poignant reminder of the flexion problems that I, and many stroke victims, have to experience to varying degrees. In my case, by using the splint and with exercises, this problem will hopefully become less with time. The fields were also showing signs of green growth but the most striking colour was yellow, in many due to the flowers of oilseed rape. I never realised what a variety of green colours were evident in the countryside at this time of year!

We had a very pleasant lunch at the garden centre and had a walk around, purchasing two plants for use in the empty pots at the front of our house. Before leaving we noticed swallows were skimming around the outbuildings of the garden centre, indicating that spring was now well underway, and on the way home we saw a large field full of sheep with lambs, one of the few flocks seen by us in our recent journeys. Perhaps this situation has been due to problems in the farming industry last year and the poor prices offered for lambs and other produce.

The major talking point at this time has been the strike of workers at the oil refinery at nearby Grangemouth, planned to start this weekend for forty-eight hours. The effect of this has been the shutdown of the plant, a secondary closure of North Sea oil pipeline production to Aberdeen, and a worry for the motorist and commercial services regarding petrol and diesel supplies and costs at the pumps. The strike is set to cause serious economic damage, if, as expected, the BP Forties pipeline is shut, cutting off £50 million each day in oil company revenue and depriving the Treasury of £30 million a day in tax. Grangemouth supplies about 30% of the UK's oil and gas and involves 1,200 workers, whose reason for striking is related to a dispute regarding pension agreements.

The Month of May Has Come!

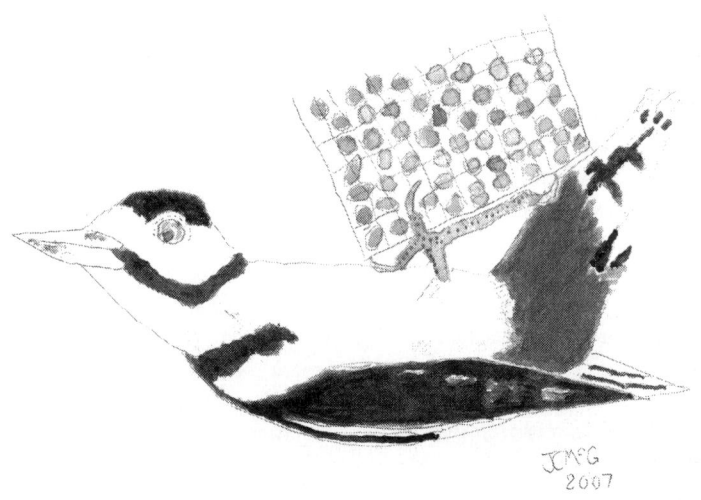

Painting of woodpecker

'Ne'er cast a clout 'til May be out.'

This is an old saying which suggests that you should not throw away winter clothes until May has been completed and refers to the appearance of new hawthorn blossom, which is said to be a true sign of the beginning of summer.

Many years ago, before I had had a chance of travelling abroad, I had a very interesting discussion on a train journey to London with a retired merchant seaman during which I asked him which of all the places he had visited he liked the most. His reply was quite unexpected! It was, 'Scotland.' Strange though it seems now to be the case, and having been very fortunate in having been to many wonderful places throughout the world, I find myself in agreement – even though it is true that given my current situation, long plane trips abroad will be less likely. The only problem with Scotland is the unpredictable weather, but once this improves with the advancing year there is no doubt that I should be able to visit a lot of places that are more convenient and just as interesting. I am encouraged by the short visits I have already made and stimulated visually by the scenery and wildlife especially. Whether this will be beneficial to my recovery or speeds up my progress remains something of an uncertainty, but to me it would seem important as well as likely. In respect of this, I can recommend a book *Scotland's Nature and Wildlife* by Kenny Taylor, which is well illustrated and contains beautiful descriptions of the Scottish countryside, wildlife, and where to find it. This book I am currently in process of reading, and it now seems to be appropriate as the month of May begins and the spring changes are now well underway.

The first day of May started cold, dull, and damp; perhaps this was why, after the dawn chorus, which began at 4.30 a.m. lasted for thirty minutes, and consisted mainly of blackbird songs, there was an almost complete silence. About three-quarters of an hour after the end of the chorus, I heard the piping triple outburst of a single song thrush over a five-minute period, possibly the same one or its mate that I had seen in a nearby garden on one of my walks. Talking about birds that I have often heard but rarely seen, during my walks I have noticed that wrens and hedge sparrows, though extremely common, are well hidden in the shrubbery and rarely venture into the open. The same can be said about the less common house sparrow, which seems to occur in sporadic small pockets around my walking area. Neither the wren or the house sparrow have not so far been seen at the garden feeding containers, though it is doubtful if wrens ever go to them anyway.

Following my visit to Astley Ainslie to be assessed for possible driving, I am due to return next week to see if, by using the original ankle splint, I can use the right foot instead of my left foot for pedal control. In view of this I propose to see how walking with it compares to walking with the battery/electrode system I have been using successfully in the last few months. In fact I walked successfully for a thirty-minute period with the splint a few days ago, and tried to see how I might be able to work with my right foot on our own car pedals. While not conclusive, this seemed to have been a helpful change.

My first outing of the day was in mid-morning, and for a change I decided to go for a walk through one of the three woodland areas nearby, both to try out the splint and see some new surroundings. The path through the woods was covered with red blaze and, though uneven in places, was a reasonable one for me to venture on. One of the first things I heard was a blackcap warbler, which I saw and identified, producing its pretty, fluting, blackbird-like song from a high branch. The wild flowers in the wood consisted of small collections of Scots bluebells and larger patches of a white acrid-smelling flower – possibly wild garlic. There were a large number of trees now producing freshly coloured green leaves, notably chestnut, hawthorn, rowan, ash, beech and sycamore, while a few rabbits scurried away ahead of me. Truly this was a magical scene, and one I had thought many months ago would for me be an extremely long way in the future, if ever! With regard to the splint, I seemed to be able to walk well enough and returned home after about thirty minutes without incident.

An interesting letter came through today's post from the Department for Work and Pensions, indicating that I was now getting a Disability Living Allowance for help with personal care and for getting around. With this I may get some financial help with regard to obtaining a car under a Motability Car Scheme, but this is something to consider once I have received a positive response from the Smart Centre and my assessment.

Tonight promised to be an interesting TV show with Glasgow Rangers playing an important semi-final football match in Italy against Fiorentina and, although I am not now a fan of Rangers and have an equal interest in rugby, I look forward to what is expected to be a great sporting night. Though it could be debated, I actually think that a top-class football match or player provides a more skilful spectacle than an equivalent rugby duel. The match was not what could be described as a feast of football brilliance but was absorbing, showed Rangers as a great defensive side. It went to extra time, with Rangers winning a deciding penalty shootout 4–2 after a goalless draw. This outstanding performance from a Scottish team means that they have reached the final of the UEFA Cup, and it is the club's first European final since 1972. It is going to be an interesting month of football, what with cup finals, close league finishes in Scotland and England, and Manchester United and Chelsea having reached the final of the Champions League of Europe earlier in the week.

During the week I had my monthly check-up visit at the GP, but since Dr Donald was not available, I was seen by a colleague, Dr Jolliffe, who checked my blood pressure. To my surprise and pleasure, the systolic (higher) value was down from last month's figure, and Dr Jolliffe said this was 'a big improvement on the original ones'. None the less there was 'still some scope for blood pressure reduction'. Accordingly, one of my tablets, doxazosin – an alpha blocker – would be increased from 2 to 4 mg per day for a trial period of two weeks to assess the results and see if any side effects occurred – early morning dizziness being one of these. At present, I now take a total of fourteen tablets each day, requiring about fifteen minutes of almost 'military-style organisation on one day each weekend with Moira's help in order to set up the next week's supply. Each packet of tablets contains a pamphlet outlining possible complications and explaining what each tablet does and why. Fortunately, so far I have not had any complications, and the medication does appear to have benefited my urological, diabetic, and blood pressure problems. One interesting and highly relevant factor that I should note is that I can no longer feel a strong, bounding pulse in my temples, which used to be the case (and was presumably an indicator of high blood pressure).

The big story at the end of the first week in May has been the major losses by Labour in the English council elections, the success of the Conservatives, and the victory of Boris Johnson over Ken Livingstone to become Mayor of London in a separate election. The latter result illustrates, I think, how public perception of a politician can be affected by voice, sense of humour and appearance, as well as important issues currently in the public domain – such as immigration, taxation, traffic congestion, housing costs, as well as the general 'lack of feeling happy'. As a plastic and cosmetic surgeon I have always had an interest in how success in life (whatever this is!) can sometimes be equated to physical appearance rather than actual abilities. How otherwise does one explain how few older women seem to be news presenters, how many women dye their hair blonde, and how both men and women seek cosmetic surgery or products, and in an increasing, if not disproportional, way? It seems very unfair but true, that if one is perceived as 'unattractive' or suffers from a disability, this will be an unhelpful feature which can only be overcome by demonstrating other exceptional qualities such as in sport, in the arts, or being a comedian!

I had another day at the end of the week trying my splint and walks as usual, in addition to a visit to another garden centre in East Lothian, where Moira and I had a very pleasant lunch and a walk round. I must admit that at the end of the afternoon I felt more tired than usual. By comparison, on the following day – Sunday – I did the same walks and had lunch at Bruntsfield Golf Club with Moira, Mr and Mrs Stuart Hamilton, their two young daughters, wore the battery-powered stimulator, and at the end of this felt much fitter! Whether this was a fair comparison or not, or due to 'one of those days' that are said to occur sometimes in a recovering stroke person, remains uncertain. The added factor of the smell of new paint in the house due to some work that had been done to the stair and banister areas may also have contributed, but by Sunday this odour was getting less. I will need to be fit for the coming week's activities, which will involve two visits to the gym, one to see the physiotherapist Julie Hooper at the McLeod Street Clinic, a visit to Astley Ainslie Hospital for further car driving assessment, and a possible trip to Inverurie at the next week end to see how Moira's mother is.

Jacki has emailed me to say that she has been home for fourteen days, having been in the Victoria Hospital for eight months, and is finding things difficult, and at times depressing as well as lonely. Unlike me of course, she has no helpful partner to be constantly available. I replied saying that it was early days yet, and Moira and I had found the care helpers extremely helpful, as was the care nurse who came later to check on how in general we were coping; this person was still to visit Jacki, and so I replied to her that things gradually get better as time goes by, and helpful assistance was almost certainly available to her if she explained what was needed. I do hope my advice will be helpful but it does illustrate how the varied problems of stroke rehabilitation for different patients with different types of stroke and home circumstances can present a real difficulty.

Walks in our garden and in the surrounding neighbourhood at this early time in May reveal increasing growth of plants and new flowers such as berberis, rhododendrons, broom, and the colourful and tropical looking, but short-lived, magnolia tree blossoms. In spite of this, I am still on the look out for honeybees – but so far without success! There are plenty of bumblebees, both white-tailed and brown, and a few wasps, but little sign of butterflies apart from one white one with orange wing tips. The new leaves are just beginning to come in the oak trees, giving them a fresh green blush, but these trees are clearly later than the majority of the other trees.

A visit to the Drumbrae gym – the first of two this week – revealed initially some disappointment, as Isla had been trans-ferred to another site and would no longer be looking after me. However, I did not need to worry, as my new instructor, Danny, seemed both keen and able to continue with exercises designed to strengthen my shoulder and right arm. He showed me a number of new techniques with regard to this.

The following day I had my follow-up review at Astley Ainslie Smart Centre, and met Sinead again. This was to see if by wearing the ankle splint I could drive using my right foot on the accelerator and my left for the brake. For this, instead of the Nissan Micra I used before, I drove around the hospital grounds in a larger Ford Focus car, and managed well enough for Sinead to say I could now go ahead and organise driving lessons! This was a great boost for me as well as Moira, and we went straight to arrange them at the recommended driving school in Edinburgh. A date in July was booked. Incidentally, as we drove out of the Smart Centre, we noticed the many beautiful pink blossomed cherry trees in grounds of the Astley Ainslie Hospital, which made a truly lovely splash of colour and must do much to raise the spirits of patients and visitors alike – especially as the day was very warm and sunny. Today was a really fine one with a temperature of 20°C in Edinburgh – let's hope it's not our summer!

In the afternoon Moira and I went to see Julie Hooper at the McLeod Street Physiotherapy Centre, the previous visit being one month ago. She felt I had definitely made progress with shoulder movements and suggested I was now ready to try the swimming pool, which should also be beneficial for my shoulder.

After such a busy day, I was happy to rest in our garden and enjoy the sunshine and watch the birds visiting the garden and the feeding containers. The stars of this were the pair of bullfinches, followed by the greenfinches, whose colours were even more impressive when viewed in the sunlight through binoculars. A further point of interest for me was the small collection of cacti which I have had for many years. Some of them are beginning to flower. They are kept in a small glass-covered building outside in our garden and had until recently been covered up with bubble wrap to protect them from any frost. It is often thought that cacti are uninteresting, unattractive, and rarely flower, but this is not what I have found. In addition they are remarkably hardy, require little care, and some of the flowering varieties are truly spectacular as well as beautiful. The range of shapes and spine colours give added interest to any collection.

One bit of good news occurred following my second visit to the gym this week the next morning: Ayla would be coming back! Thus we can renew the 'team'. Danny still showed me some more useful exercises and I did five minutes on the bicycle at a higher setting and managed this well. He himself was being transferred to another centre in Leith, and I would not get him again; this seems to be fairly normal for these leisure centres. The weather again was surprisingly good again with hardly a cloud in the sky, and I went for my usual walks enjoying the summery weather. For the first time I heard the sounds of very young nestlings coming from high up in the roof margins of some of the houses – probably starlings. Although I saw blue tits flying in and out of the garden nest box, all was quiet as yet. I was kept amused during the afternoon watching my granddaughter, Holly, toddling about in our garden and learning to fall in and out of various cars and trucks. She has started to say a few words and seems to understand a few more like 'biscuit', 'milk', and 'bye'.

At the weekend Moira and I went up to see Moira's mother in

Inverurie, Aberdeenshire, and stayed overnight in the Strathburn Hotel as we had done in March. Once again, we had a good time and saw Ron, Edna, Norman, Sheila, and Moira's mother for an evening meal. I enjoyed all of this trip including the journey and seeing the countryside in its springtime clothes. In addition to the various shades and textures of green, the new exciting colour seemed to be yellow – again in various shades, from the rich fields of rapeseed and the golden-yellow patches of gorse at the side of the roads and fields, to the starry collections of the many dandelions that lined the road verges. Of these, the gorse was the most spectacular and widespread. According to an old country saying, 'While the gorse is in flower, Britain will never be conquered.' Gorse is an excellent fuel and burns fiercely, causing heath fires to spread rapidly. It is often planted as a hedge or as a windbreak for livestock. The last of the daffodil patches at the entrance to Aberdeen gave a little colour, but the majority of these were now passed their best and their presence was only seen by rows of dead heads on their stems like some defeated army. A striking new colour, not noticed before, was due to the recent emergence of copper beech trees and their rich brown colour – much less common than the soft light green ordinary beech trees, also just coming into leaf. Some large trees had still not come out with leaves, and in some of these colonies of rooks could be seen nesting, particularly in areas where there were a group of similar trees, either beeches or elms. I wondered whether the rooks chose certain types of trees because of their size and grouping, or because of the later leaf production in these species. Another point to ponder on was the apparent quietness following the recent fuel crisis and the problems caused by the recent forty-eight-hour strike at Grangemouth; certainly there were plenty of cars on the road and no shortage of fuel at the pumps. Perhaps the issues have been resolved, but whatever happens it will not bother the rooks!

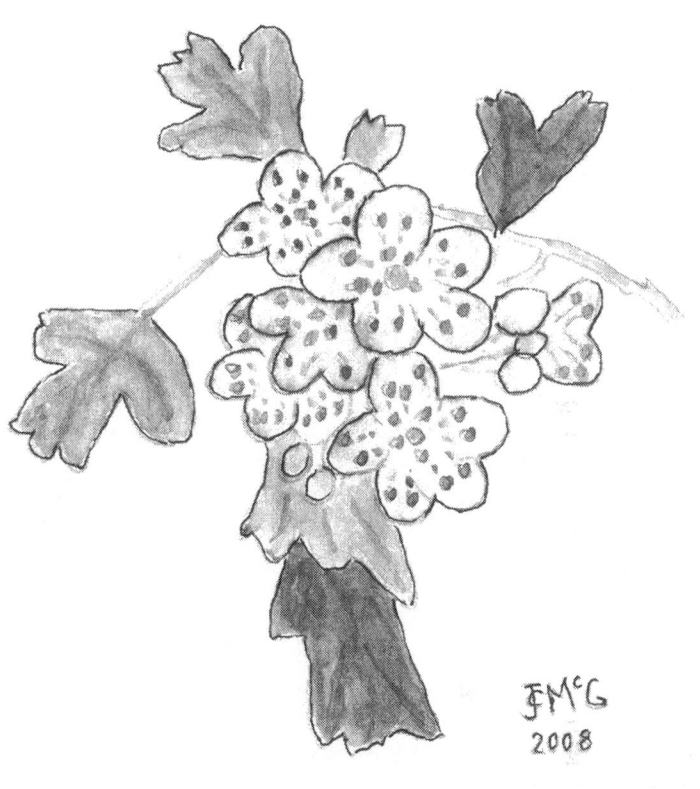

JMcG
2008

HAWTHORN BLOSSOM

May Continues and the Hawthorn Blossom Breaks Out!

It is now nearly fourteen days into May, and luckily each day seems to pass quickly and be of interest. The early weeks have been warmer than usual and there has been less rain than last year, according to the weather forecasters. There have been major events this month elsewhere in the world, which put any problems that I might think I have into perspective: a large cyclone destroying large areas of Burma occurred in early May, causing many thousands of deaths and not alleviated by the military leaders of that secretive country, who seemed to prevent aid workers from entering to help distribute aid. As if that was not enough, there has been a major earthquake in the centre of China which, the first since the 1970s, has destroyed many buildings and killed thousands, including school children. As in the Burmese situation, the final death toll may never be known and may be numbered in tens of thousands or more. It has been estimated that in China a total of five million people have been made homeless.

This week I am due to visit the GP again for my blood pressure check, and the stroke nurse has sent a card indicating she will be visiting to see how we are coping. I also have to visit the swimming pool at Drumbrae at the end of the week, which will be a new and stressful experience, no doubt!

The visit to see Dr Jolliffe went well – my blood pressure measurement was satisfactory and both measurements were down on the previous levels. On the basis that it could be lowered a little more and thus far I had had no dizzy spells, the dose of doxazosin could be doubled, and this might bring the levels close to the normal values for my age. A further appointment was made for two weeks to be reassessed. There was also a home visit from the stroke nurse – Sheila Forsyth – which really was to let her know how things were and how we were managing. She was pleased to record that my blood pressure was down to about half the original levels nine months ago, and was close to the value that Professor Dennis had wished I should attain.

I had, of course, let the Driver and Vehicle Licensing Agency (DVLA) know about my stroke, and in particular the Drivers' Medical Group were also informed, as I wished to resume driving again. A series of forms were sent by the latter for me to complete and send back within three weeks, and included a consent form for me to agree for medical information to be obtained from any of the doctors involved in my care. The forms were completed and sent back in forty-eight hours.

There was an interesting discussion on the early morning BBC TV programme on the possible value of listening to a half-hour of music – preferably quiet – in reducing stress and lowering blood pressure when it was 'slightly' raised. While this seemed possible, there has been no strong evidence as yet that this method works to reduce very high blood pressure. Similar stimulation of other senses, such as by aromatherapy or by painting or by watching nature or even fish in ponds or tanks, might also be effective. It has also been shown that visits of dogs and other pets to ward patients can also reduce stress, and the mere stroking of these also has a lowering effect on the blood pressure. It is interesting that I remember once or twice seeing a lady and a red setter visiting the ward for this very purpose. While the value of all of these factors may not be scientifically proven, it would seem that all of them could be helpful in stroke prevention and management, in addition to diet, medication and exercise.

Whether watching exciting sporting events is actually 'non-stressful' or not is also a matter for debate, and there has been some evidence that blood pressure can be raised during such events. However, overall there can be a good feeling among the supporters of a successful team which can be translated into the workforce and general increased output. Presumably, the reverse will be true! Over the next few weeks of May this will be tested with the climax of relegations, league winners, and cup winners in the football scene, in the local arena and in this year, the European one.

The first of these football occasions was the final of the UEFA Cup in Manchester between Glasgow Rangers and a relatively unknown team from Russia called Zenit St Petersburg. After a fairly poor game, Zenit, who were the better attacking team, deservedly won by two goals to nil. It was said that over 100,000 Rangers fans were in Manchester, though only a lesser number had tickets and got into the stadium to see the game; many of the rest watched the game on specially arranged large screens in outside areas. The only problem was that in one site, the screen failed to work, causing unrest and stress and a resulting violent confrontation between the police and the supporters, which has spoiled what had up to this match been an unblemished record of good behaviour in the tournament. There were several arrests, and one Zenit supporter was stabbed. The mess of cans and other waste material left behind in the streets by the supporters after the match was also a sad but not unexpected outcome of this large event. The supporters blame the police for overreacting, and the police maintain they acted reasonably in trying to control a small minority of troublemakers! This is undoubtedly the downside of football as a sport and one aspect that happens rarely, if at all, in others such as golf, tennis, horse racing, snooker, or rugby.

As anticipated, I went with Moira to try the swimming pool at the Drumbrae Leisure Centre. We found excellent facilities here, including a large disabled persons' room for changing, and helpful assistance provided by the pool staff in order to get into the water, including the use of a special hoist seat to lift me in as well as out. The increased buoyancy provided by the water certainly gave me the possibility of exercising both my legs and shoulders, as Julie had predicted, and I intend to add this to my rehabilitation programme. An added positive result of this visit was that we met up with Lenny and his wife, May, and another stroke man, Jim, and his wife, Betty, when we were able to discuss matters of mutual interest. This, I believe, will be a major help for all of us and will offer the great advantage of providing a social network of support for the wives as well as those affected.

An article in the local paper (the *Evening News*) of Thursday, 15 May by Gareth Rose caught my eye, and should be of great interest for stroke patients. In the Astley Ainslie Hospital a patient persuaded her former employers to donate a Wii games console to the gym and occupational departments. Both these departments indicate that the Wii will be of great value for hand–eye coordination and balance, and can used sitting or standing and for stroke, brain injuries, and other neurological conditions such as multiple sclerosis and Guillain-Barré syndrome. Not only can it be used therapeutically, but it is an enjoyable activity that can increase engagement of the patient with rehabilitation. It can be used to play boxing, bowling, tennis, and golf.

A neighbour's house alarm went off unexpectedly at 5 a.m. during the week, and Moira and another neighbour went in to turn the alarm off and check there had been no break-in. Why it went off seemed to be a mystery until a possible and surprising explanation presented itself when we investigated curious tapping sounds coming from one of our own back rooms – these were caused by a number of jackdaws! Why they were tapping on the windows was unknown, but it seemed possible that they were doing the same in the neighbour's house, thereby setting off the alarm by their vibrations. A gang of marauding jackdaws are now visiting our feeding station and rapidly depleting the supplies – something that had not happened in previous times, and was preventing the smaller birds from feeding. Since jackdaws are usually found near old ruined buildings or cliffs, there occurrence in our area seems very strange. We will try to reduce this problem by looking for a different style of feeding container.

The middle weekend of this month started with an evening out on the Friday night as guest of Mr Pradip Datta at one of his favourite dining-out spots – The Railbridge in South Queensferry – where we had an excellent meal and enjoyed the stunning views of the rail and the road bridges over the Forth. Pradip was a superb and talkative host, and Moira and I had a truly morale-boosting experience. As a former honorary secretary of the Royal College of Surgeons of Edinburgh, and current Council Member, he remains a loyal friend and an example of all that has been good to me as a member of the same College. As a gift, I was given by him a bottle of the single malt whisky – Old Pulteney – produced locally in his adopted home town of Wick in the far north of Scotland, and which I will greatly enjoy and treasure!

With regard to the jackdaw problem, though I have no objection to these interesting and very intelligent birds, they are clearly causing problems and grab the majority of the nuts, as well as frightening the smaller birds away. Moira and I went out to the nearby garden centre in West Lothian, had a very satisfactory lunch, and purchased two new bird feeder containers, one for nuts and the other for seeds. Both were surrounded by an outside cage which would allow small but not larger birds to pass through. The manufacturers – 'The Nuttery' – gave a guarantee of their being long lasting and not allowing squirrels and larger birds to pass through, ensuring that smaller birds have access to feed in safety. Time will tell if this is in fact true.

To complete this weekend, Moira drove me to one of my favourite places in Scotland to see my cousin Lynne, her husband Alan, and my aunt May at their farm, 'Killymingan', near Kirkgunzeon in Dumfriesshire. We went along the picturesque route through Biggar and returned by the different but equally stunning scenic Moffat and the 'Devil's Elbow' back to Edinburgh. In contrast to our recent visit to Aberdeenshire, I noticed some differences in the farming and flora. Firstly, there were many fields with sheep and plenty of lambs, a few herds of dairy cattle, no fields with crops such as yellow rapeseed, and much less gorse growth. According to Alan, the fields are less arable than in Fife or Aberdeenshire. The moorlands and the rolling hills were quite different from the more jagged and awesome mountains in the Grampians, and lacked the purple tinges of heather and the herds of deer. Evidence of forestry work was seen frequently, both with planting and with vast areas laid bare by deliberate cutting down. The second difference seemed to be that the colour white seemed to predominate in the countryside, with the pale sparkling of many blooming hawthorn trees and shrubs, the candelabra-like flowers of the chestnut trees, white wild hemlock-like flowers at the roadsides, and the feathery pale white dandelion 'seed clocks'.

Moira and I were treated to a splendid farmhouse lunch of soup, bread, and cheese and sat at a window looking out at a well-kept garden and a panoramic view of farmland and distant hills – a truly spectacular site, and one that everyone enjoys. There is now much more of a wide vista because of the need to cut down an aged and spectacular elm tree as a result of Dutch elm disease. Outside, a bird feeder filled with peanuts was busily 'attacked' by voracious house sparrows who lived in the nearby ivy-clad walls of an old cowshed. No other types of birds were seen, probably frightened away by the noisy yet amusing sparrows – quite a contrast from our own garden feeders, where so far no sparrows have been seen. Aunt May, although not a direct relative of mine, had herself suffered a stroke or strokes within the last few years, which affected her ability to speak clearly. However, she was able to communicate well using a writing pad and stayed herself in the farm, receiving help from community care and her daughters – one of whom, Lynne, lives nearby and can look in every day.

My walks around the area of our house still continued at about thirty minutes twice each day, and possibly because I had a cold – the first I have had for almost nine months – I have not quite felt so fit. It might be related to the increased medication which I had started recently. There were no episodes of dizziness The gardens were becoming steadily more colourful, with new flowers such as azaleas, primulas, tulips, clematis, lilacs, and laburnum trees, with their long chains of golden-yellow flowers which have earned the tree the name of 'golden rain'. The coming week promised to be a quieter one for me, with only one gym visit, but I still planned to work at my exercises, especially with my shoulder and hand.

The Last Few Weeks of May

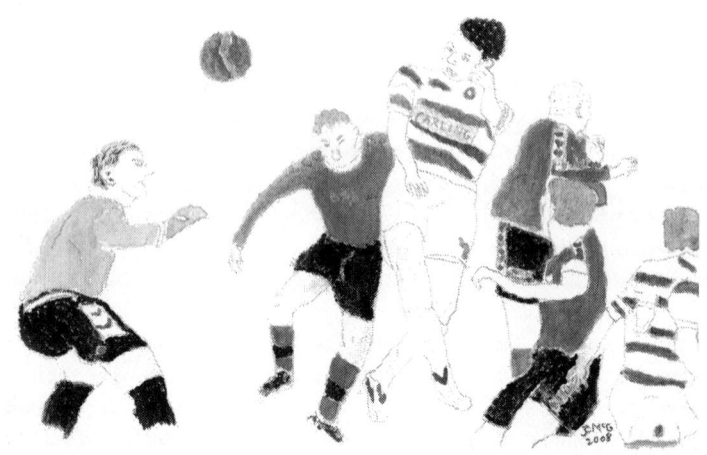

The week beginning 19 May began dry and colder but promised to be very interesting because of various football matches, including the Scottish Cup, the Champions League Final of Europe between Manchester United and Chelsea, and the cliff-hanging final matches involving Rangers and Celtic to decide the winner of the Premier Scottish League Championship. Why has rugby struggled professionally in Scotland, and why did the Rugby Cup at Murrayfield Stadium at the beginning of May – won by Melrose, who defeated Heriots – only attract a crowd of 6,000 people? Far fewer attend club matches. School rugby was undoubtedly a major reason in my own life for the great friend-ships which were established between parents and the sons they watched playing throughout their time at school and thereafter – hence 'the Rugby Crowd'. Senior rugby is less attractive for me, though I still watch it avidly on television. The rules are difficult to understand and the possibility for serious injury is greater than in football. Rugby is still largely a sport to be found in the private schools, and the opportunities to play soccer are more widely available to the young boys and girls, as well as being easier to play, with minimal set-up. Perhaps these are the reasons for football to be more popular sport in Scotland. Manchester United won after extra time and a penalty shoot-out – very good entertainment, especially if one is neutral or a United supporter!

I had a bad night after this and felt I hardly slept; I seemed to cough a lot, which also upset Moira. However, I still was able to do my usual morning walk and felt well doing this. Again I had no dizziness, and hopefully the additional medication was reducing my blood pressure without producing unhelpful side effects; next week's check-up with the GP should provide the proof or not.

The new bird feeders certainly seem to have stopped the jack-daw visits, but now the only birds coming to the feeders appear to be tits and even then there are many fewer than before. The blue tits are regularly going in and out of the nest box, but so far there are no sounds of any chicks.

Celtic defeated Dundee United, while simultaneously Rangers were defeated by Aberdeen and consequently Celtic became the 2008 League Champions – for the third year in succession. Rangers have now only the Cup Final to look forward to in two days' time to give their supporters something sing about! At least one half of the Glasgow supporters will be happy over the summer months, and their work production will probably be better than otherwise it might have been; such is the power of sport and psychology.

Image and success in the media and on the political scene seem to me to be closely linked in a way to how people are perceived, and support for or against is similar to the effect of either being a successful sportsperson or supporting a successful team or hero. The current seemingly everlasting American Presidential nomination elections are a point in question, as is the diminishing belief in the current leadership of the Labour Party in Britain, particularly when contrasted with the previous leader, even given his decisions in overseas activities. It is for these reasons that I think that everyone who has an acquired or birth defect should be given the best opportunity to obtain the best image possible; but they themselves must play their part and make every effort to improve themselves by having their own personal goals to aim for. Failing this, there is a need for our society to become more aware and caring of those less fortunate in appearance as well as function. At the same time it is evident that more and more money is being spent on anti-ageing and beautification surgery and materials. Whether this is a good thing or not remains to be seen but it is not necessarily of immediate benefit to the less fortunate.

Rangers managed to defeat Queen of the South by three goals to two in a very interesting Scottish Cup Final, in which the underdog First Division side gave an excellent account of themselves, while Rangers managed to salvage something from what has been a hard and testing season. Football this month has been of considerable interest to the British public, with plenty of interest and controversy to stimulate their senses. It made me think about achievement and team effort, and coupled with my newly found interest in artwork, I produced a painting based on a newspaper photograph of the Celtic player, with the unusual name Vennegoor of Hesselink, scoring a headed goal against Dundee United in the last game of the season – a goal which effectively won the League Championship from their close rival, Rangers. Prior to this match both teams were equal on points, though Celtic had a better goal difference. Rangers actually lost their final match, played at the same time against Aberdeen. I hope that the painting does some sort of justice to what that sporting occasion merited and the effort of the player concerned. Unfortunately, the Edinburgh team that I have followed for many years has not done so well – nor has the other one!

The weekend television had the annual spectacle of the *Eurovision Song Contest*, in which the British entry came equal last! Clearly, the voting was distinctly political and 'neighbourly', not based on musical content, and the more gimmicks and scantily clad extras, the better for obtaining votes. None the less, I admit to having watched the show to the bitter end, probably along with many other sad souls! There are several much more interesting and probably more balanced programmes this week coming on television, which I am looking forward to, including *Springwatch* and *Britain's Got Talent*. The first of these is a nature programme, partly live, and the latter will be a live nightly semi-final competition exhibiting various British people showing a remarkable array of talents. The eventual winner, chosen by public telephone votes, gets the honour of appearing at this year's Royal Variety Show in front of a member of the Royal Family; and presumably, even for some of the losers, the nationwide exposure can result in new careers.

At the weekend, Moira and I took what we termed 'a trial car run' to East Kilbride and Cathcart Golf Club, in view of our invitation to attend a 40th Wedding Anniversary celebration of one of our oldest friends, Jean and Graham, at the end of June. It was a very pleasant day weather-wise, but spoiled somewhat by delays on the way caused by an accident on the main road into Edinburgh. However, it did mean a very picturesque journey home through Winchburgh and Kirkliston, along a road less well known but very quiet – one which I had frequently used when I was working.

The weather in Scotland has been much sunnier and drier than in the southern parts of Britain and my cold seems to be easing. Certainly, I have been able to do my thirty-minute walks without any problems and no dizziness. Tomorrow I will be seen by the GP and it will be seen whether the new medication has brought my blood pressure down to safe and sensible levels. A new chair has been delivered, and this should help both posture as well as comfort. This chair is a single motor electric riser-recliner model that we purchased on the advice of the Disabled Living Centre at the Smart Centre from Med-Ecosse Ltd, based at Loanhead near Edinburgh.

Moira and I visited the Royal Botanic Gardens in Edinburgh on what turned out to be a rather cold and windy afternoon, but it gave me a good walk which also involved climbing up some reasonable inclines. I felt very pleased about yet another 'achievement' towards my recovery, as well as seeing the beautiful display of colourful azaleas. Because of concern about a new fungal disease that has killed oaks in America and has been found in some plants in the UK – but not yet in oaks – we went in and out over chemically treated mats.

Another interesting account from a stroke victim was published in the *Scottish Daily Mail* on 27 May, adapted from a personal account of a fifty-six-year-old head teacher: 'The moment my world imploded', by Martin Stephen. It is worthy of comment in that it illustrates a different type of stroke than mine, a much quicker early recovery, a very short inpatient stay, and a return to work after eight weeks with evidently little serious residual disability. However, his account illustrates his determination and character in the face of what was obviously a very life-shattering experience. Every stroke has different causes and effects but, although recovery may be unpredictable in time as well as extent, there is an optimism which his account projects, and hopefully mine does too! I am realistic enough to know I will never be able to return to my work as a surgeon, but this does not worry me at my stage in life. I am happy enough to have survived and to have made the recovery I have to date.

The visit to the GP was very satisfactory with my blood pressure of 144/64 – apparently close to a figure that should keep me alive and healthy, although I wondered if the diastolic lower value was too low. There was to be no change in medication, and it was felt that I was looking well and 'seemed to be moving better'. The visit to the gym the next day was a little worrying in that I only managed two five-minute turns on the bicycle, although I managed to complete the various shoulder and thigh exercises without difficulty. I will put this down to my cold, which is still evident. Certainly, I was able to manage my usual thirty-minute walks, though not so swiftly. The following day Moira took me to the Leisure Centre swimming pool where I spent thirty minutes or so moving my legs and shoulder in the increased buoyancy provided by the water. Moira decided to join the Leisure Centre, so she will now be able to use the facilities of the pool and gym at the same time as me if she wishes. We met up in the waiting area with Lenny, May, and Jim's wife, Betty, and this enabled useful exchange of information and discussion about various problems encountered in hospital and after discharge home. For example, we were able to tell Betty that her husband was still entitled to a bus pass, and we all learned from Betty about a book and key available for information and use all over Britain for disabled persons' toilets! We also agreed to meet for a 'get together' and meal in about ten day's time.

The final day of May was very warm with a temperature of 23–25° Centigrade, as measured for outside temperature by our car. The morning walk was very hot but pleasant, and for the first time this year I saw a honeybee at a nearby bush of broom, along with several bumblebees. The blooms have long since left the cherry trees and lie in the gutters and driveways, dried up, their colourful red and pink flowers now only a memory of early May. Instead, the new bright colour is provided by the yellow laburnum trees that are a frequent sight in the various gardens, and the variable colours of azaleas and dwarf rhododendrons. The heaths in our front garden, so long in bloom and very colourful, are now in decline, as their flowers are withered and brown. Sadly, there is still no evidence of blue tit activities in the garden nest box.

Tonight promises to be quite interesting on the TV with the finals of talent shows. On BBC the winner who will become 'Nancy' in a London West End production of *Oliver!*, while ITV has a show of Britain's best talents, the winner of which will have a place on this year's Royal Variety Show. The winners, selected by viewer's votes on the night, are also guaranteed a lucrative career, and the runners-up may also achieve their own personal aims through their wide exposure on TV. Although I did not see the game on TV, over 80,000 people attended the Rugby Union championship decider in England between Wasps and Leicester, which suggests that in contrast to Scotland, rugby does in fact have a large support south of the border. Similarly, in middle England, rugby league has a very large following, and this does not feature in Scotland. This may be one of the reasons why soccer remains the main team game followed, and less money is available for rugby in Scotland.

The winners of the two TV programmes, which apparently attracted several million viewers, represented what might be termed 'true British grit' in that Jodie Prenger, who won the 'Nancy' competition, had lost several stones in weight intention-ally before entering, and the fourteen-year-old boy, George Sampson, who won the talent show with a stunning break-dance routine and had failed in a previous attempt the previous year, started in competitions against thousands of entrants. Although this was very impressive, I was even more impressed by the TV programme the night before which also demonstrated true grit in adversity, in which ten young people with various physical and mental disabilities managed to complete a challenging crossing of the Andes!

What does this show me? It demonstrates what can be achieved against the odds – let's hope I don't let myself down!

Incidentally, the Met Office reported that May was the warmest May ever recorded in Scotland, was the eighth sunniest May, and the eighteenth sunniest month overall since records began at the start of the First World War.

Flaming June?

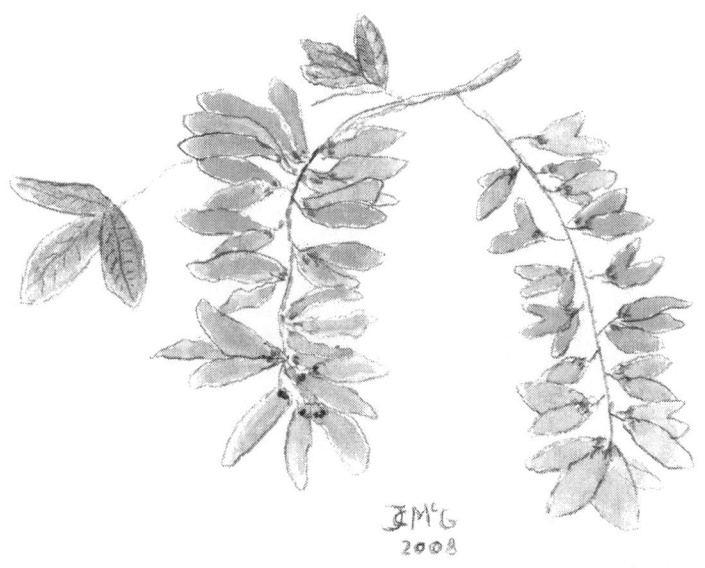

Painting of laburnum flower

The first day of June was decidedly a gloomy, wet affair and contrasted greatly with what had occurred during most of May and the day before. Moira and I decided to go to the morning church service, which also happened to be the Church of Scotland Communion Service at the Cramond Kirk. The service was conducted by the Reverend Dr Russell Barr, our minister, who had visited me several times both in and outwith my stay in hospital. His excellent approach and warm support for me and Moira were greatly appreciated. I was pleased that I was able to manage to stay the course of the service, including being able to sit down and stand up when required, although my right shoulder still ached. It was too wet for me to go out, and so for the first day since I started walking myself outside I did not go out walking. I still was able to do my shoulder exercises inside, as I was now used to doing every night before going to bed.

The next day was dull but dry, and so I was able to go on my walks. The laburnum trees continue to brighten up the gardens nearby and this prompted me to try to draw and paint it as well as read about it. The seed pods are poisonous and children should be warned about confusing these with peas when they ripen in July and August. The tree has been in Britain for more than 300 years and comes originally from Central and Southern Europe. Strangely, it has not established itself outwith the suburban gardens in spite of the abundance of seeds produced. The dark wood is hard and enduring. It has been used as a substitute for ebony and for making musical instruments, by wood turners, and cabinetmakers. A member of the pea and bean family, it is actually very closely related to the common broom.

My walk in the evening was very pleasant around the local roads, although towards the end I seemed to drag my right foot a little – a battery change for my foot stimulator seemed to be in order. The predominant birdsong was now coming from numerous blackbirds, many singing from the tops of houses and often television aerials; presumably all were now settled in their territories and with partners with nests. These birds were also now the main singers in the hour-long dawn chorus, which was beginning at about 3.30 a.m.! A song thrush still sang during the dawn as well as late at night just as darkness was falling at about 11 p.m., even when the blackbirds had stopped – as if to say, 'you may outnumber me but I can outlast you all'!

A visit to Edinburgh Zoo was undertaken midweek during a sunny afternoon and proved to be an interesting and physically challenging experience, particularly as there are many hills to climb as well as descend. In fact it did not appear to me at this visit that facilities for those requiring wheelchairs or with a walking disability were helpful to this group of visitors. Moira and I were fortunate that, as a life member, it got me in free, as was our car parking, and furthermore, Moira got in free as a 'carer' for me! We also were able to enter and exit using a special members' gate situated about halfway up the zoo and at the top end of the car park. Moira, very wisely, took the wheelchair along for use during part of the visit, but only used it on the level parts when I needed to have a rest. She found it impossible to push me up or down any of the frequent and sometimes very steep slopes, but it gave me practice in walking! Obviously we were limited at this visit as to what we could travel to see, but I thoroughly enjoyed seeing the penguins, the long-limbed monkeys swinging on high, and the rainbow lorikeets – all beautifully presented in large enclosed areas. Unfortunately, there was no possibility of feeding nectar to the free-flying colourful lorikeets, which was something I and the visitors had looked forward to; but for some reason was not allowed at this time, although it had been permitted in the past. After a nice ice cream and a very pleasant visit lasting about two hours we left for home.

During this first week of June I found I could tie my short trouser tape using my right hand and zip up my sweater. These seem to be small accomplishments but represented a step forward for me! At the gym, Ayla was off sick, but Moira, helped by one of the other staff members, was able to take me through the various exercises. The following day we went to the swimming pool and Moira came in with me, although she herself was extremely uncertain about her ability to swim; she kept in the shallows! This was now my second visit to the pool, and certainly I was getting more confident and exercising my legs and shoulder to good advantage in the water. It will be interesting to see when I am assessed by Julie Hooper at the start of next week if I have improved in any way. I find it quite difficult to know but I certainly have not gone backwards. I am quite resigned to the fact that recovery of my arm and shoulder will be slow as well as unpredictable, even though I find it extremely frustrating.

I continue each night to try to undertake exercises suggested by Julie, with or without Moira's keen supervision.

A seat in our back garden watching Holly potter about proved very interesting, in that one of our recent mysteries was solved. The cause of the recent 'window tapping' was seen to be a crow and not the jackdaws. The culprit was observed attacking a neighbour's window, possibly thinking a reflection was a rival bird! At the same time a blue tit was seen going into the nest box approximately every two minutes, but I could hear no sounds of any chicks as yet. The numbers of birds attending the new feeders was definitely down and tits were now the most common visitors. One jackdaw came but did not try to feed. In late afternoon I was pleased to see a woodpecker, who appeared to feed successfully though its visit was very brief.

At the end of the week, on the Friday, Moira and I met up with Lenny, Jim, and their wives for the planned get-together evening meal, which we had at The Harp in Corstorphine. This proved to be very pleasant and the food was good. We had promised not to talk about strokes, and for the most part we achieved this, but I felt the contact with others who had had similar major changes to their lives and that of our wives was a most useful thing for all concerned.

A minor crisis occurred during the first weekend with the foot pressure connector and the insole, which kept coming apart when I was walking which, of course, interrupted the circuit for walking well. It was solved by using a new insole put on top of the old one that had become worn, and the adhesive had also failed. Moira came with me on my first walk with the new insole to verify that this new arrangement worked as it did. A new toy for me to play with – a pedometer – was also purchased and, once I have worked out how it works, it will give me something more to use to help estimate the different distances on the various walks that I do around where I live.

On the Sunday, Moira and I had lunch at the Bruntsfield Golf Club with our friends Niall and Agnes, and an enjoyable time was had by all. Niall promised to take me out in his golf buggy in about a week's time around the golf course, when perhaps I could try putting and chipping. This again would be something that I looked forward to and represented an important stage in my recovery process.

The visit to see Julie Hooper raised my spirits further by her approach and attitude. I was able to tell her about my visits to the gym and swimming pool. She had some new and useful sugges-tions regarding exercises I should try to improve my foot and ankle at home as well as in the pool. She was happy that I was still doing the shoulder exercises and thought my mobility was improving, albeit slowly. She was also careful to advise that I should not be causing any pain, 'though discomfort would be expected'.

My walks at this time were conducted more confidently because the insole problem seemed to have been solved and my cold was gone. It was just as well, because the wind had become more of an issue and I had to be more alert and probably more physically active than I had had to be in the recent weeks. The weather was still dry and warm.

Coincidentally, there was an interesting programme on BBC TV called *Britain Under Water* examining why last summer's floods, which occurred in June and July last year mainly in Southern England and Hull, had been so devastating. They were the worst for 150 years, and amounted to the most serious civil disaster in the UK since World War II. They were probably related to a freak weather situation involving a downward shift of an Atlantic jet stream during these months. The serious results with regard to properties flooded and families forced to live in cramped temporary accommodation were shown and discussed. It put my stroke and its results into some perspective!

With regard to this, a further unwelcome news item appeared this week – 9 June – three young soldiers had been killed in action in Afghanistan, making a total of 100 killed since 2001. One of these young soldiers came from Dumfries, and their ages ranged from nineteen to twenty-two years – a terrible loss for them and their families.

On a happier note, I have greatly enjoyed watching *Spring-watch 2008* on BBC 2, hosted by Bill Oddie, helped by Kate Humble and Simon King based in the Cairngorms. The main base was in Norfolk, so there was much on the wildlife in the reed beds and water areas, wonderful views of nests and fledge-lings, and excellent educational content delivered in a humorous yet interesting manner. I liked the contribution of Simon – always enthusiastic no matter where he is and what the weather is like! Of particular note were the almost unique views of the Scottish wild cat, the goldeneye duck chicks jumping from their nest box onto the ground below, the crested tits, the capercaillies, the ospreys, the dawn sounds and the beautiful scenery The programme is for the most part live, and is over three weeks except Fridays, Saturdays, and Sundays. Clearly, there must be a large back-up of other cameras and other individuals who contribute to the success of this popular subject, so teamwork is essential for success. I learned for the first time about the charming little dotterel, whose eggs and chicks are solely looked after by the duller male and breeds on the barren mountains in north and west of Britain – a good advert for women's lib!

From the sport point of view, rugby internationals for Scotland in Argentina, Ireland in New Zealand, and Wales in South Africa, the start of the European football championship and the start of the grass court tennis championships at Queen's Club in London, culminating in Wimbledon in a fortnight's time, all occur during this month. The disappointing thing this week was that the rugby teams lost their first matches, none of the UK countries qualified to take part in the football tournament, and Lewis Hamilton, our new British hope, failed miserably to finish in the Canadian Formula 1 racing car championship race! Still, there was the hope that Andy Murray of Scotland would fulfil his early promise on the tennis courts!

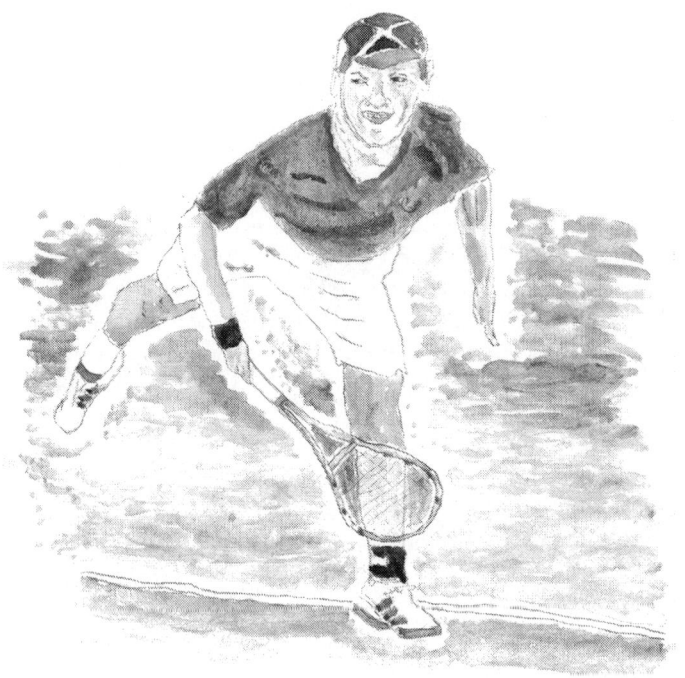

MURRAY

JCMcG
2008

The Sport in June – Mine as Well!

A question which has interested me and countless other fans of tennis, is why Britain has for many years been unable to produce a male or female Wimbledon champion? Countries like Serbia, Spain, Switzerland, and Russia currently seem to have been able to produce excellent champions – so what has been the problem? Are the tennis players in Britain too spoiled and not motivated to be fit and practise enough compared to those in other countries? Is there too much competition with regard to other sports that might be available for the youngsters to take up? Will the great new hope – Andy Murray – be able to achieve success? I do not know, but the next few weeks will be very interesting!

During this, the second week in June, I went to the gym and the swimming pool to build on my various exercises. Ayla was unavailable but I was supervised by Euan, who showed me some new things to try including the walking treadmill, a vibrating apparatus, and a thigh-strengthening machine. I went home sore but happy! When I got back home I was delighted to see an email from my last NHS secretary, Linda, in St John's Hospital in West Lothian. In it she asked how I and the family were doing and sent her best wishes, along with those of ward staff and other colleagues. This was a particularly pleasing message to receive and, at this time in my recovery, one which illustrates the commitment and loyalty of the staff in my former main work-place. I replied indicating my thanks and suggesting I might come and visit at a mutually convenient time – naturally Moira would have to take me. Two other messages came simultaneously and were also morale-boosting. The first of these was a request to review a submitted article to the *Journal of Plastic Reconstructive and Aesthetic Surgery*, and the second was from Professor Burd, the current Editor, who thanked me for my contributions to the journal and also confirmed that my most recent submitted article would be published 'soon'.

It is nearly halfway through June and almost one month to go to 'celebrate' my one year after the onset of my stroke! I certainly feel that my life and that of Moira's has been changed unexpectedly and significantly. Looking back, I am surprised at how we have coped, and at this point, what has been achieved in spite of what now seems to have been a horrendous experience, though at each stage this did not feel to be too bad. Does this reflect on the excellent care as well as advice that I have had, the support of my wife and family, my own determination, or good luck? Perhaps all of these have played a part, but the main thing is – I am still here and able to live a happy life!

I think that the care for strokes – at least in the Edinburgh area – is a tribute to the NHS. As it happens, the NHS came into existence on 5 July 1948 and will celebrate its sixtieth anniversary next month. It offered a free service to the entire population of the United Kingdom and was the first such offered in the Western world. The founder of this was the then Health Minister, Aneurin Bevan, who said, 'Not only is it available to the whole population freely, but it is intended… to generalise the best health service advice and treatment.' I am not sure, however, if given the tremendous new pressures of the ageing population, the new expensive procedures and drugs, the requests of patients, and the recent influx of people from the European Community countries, this type of service can continue without modification. I am also not certain that as far as the care of strokes are concerned, the same degree of excellent care that I have received is available throughout Scotland, as well as Britain, but it is something that must be aimed for.

My new toy – the distance and step counter – proved to be extremely interesting, and certainly it gives me something extra to make my daily walks more meaningful. For all my usual walks I can now get some idea of the distances covered. Most of the walks are for at least half a mile, while the longest measured as yet is just over one mile. Wearing the ankle splint as opposed to wearing the electrical stimulator seemed to be equally as helpful, and this is reassuring in case the latter does not work for any reason. Walking in windy conditions or downhill appeared to require more steps, as might be expected from the feeling I had of more physical effort required in these situations.

Betty, wife of Jim, telephoned on Saturday morning, 14 June, to ask if Moira and I would like to join them in a visit to a local park – the St Margaret Park in Corstorphine – where Jim often went to walk, but we had never actually been. We went round to their house and travelled in their car the short distance to the park, and I accompanied Jim in a walk which involved going round a roughly quadrilateral pathway several times – the measured distance according to my measurer being just over one mile approximately, and in my case 2,253 steps! This was in fact the greatest recorded non-stop distance thus far I had walked since my stroke. Of great interest to me was how well Moira and Betty appeared to be getting on with sharing both experiences and ideas.

In the early afternoon after the walk in the park, Moira and I decided to go for lunch to the garden centre in West Lothian on what was a cold but sunny day. This was a convenient place we have visited on several occasions and always enjoyed the meal and environment. The short car journey and return through mainly rural farmlands gives nice views of Fife, the Forth, and the two impressive bridges across the Forth. It was striking that the grass and wild flowers at the roadside were now profuse and wild, with hemlock-like white flowers, buttercups, and tall white ox-eye daisies predominating. Apart from occasional patches of broom, yellow was a rare colour, and the golden gorse and the brilliant white snow-like areas of the hawthorn bushes were now gone having changed into shrivelled brown flower remnants.

The following day – Father's Day – was a dull but dry one. I was given a nice card and a mug with photographs of my three grandchildren on the side. Moira and I went with Trudy, Callum and Holly to visit the Botanic Gardens, where we had lunch in the cafeteria and admired the beautiful memorial gardens dedicated to the Queen Mother close to the North Gate. I watched a very enthralling tennis final on BBC 2 television in the afternoon – the Stella Artois grass court final in London at Queen's Club between Nadal and Djokovich, which the former won. From what I saw it is very doubtful if any British player, including our Andy Murray, can offer a realistic hope at the Wimbledon Championships due in about nine days. It demonstrated the fitness and skill required to be a champion and the popularity of tennis as a sport in this country. Here I must confess that my secret ambition as a boy, after wanting to be a plastic surgeon, was that I would have liked to have competed at Wimbledon and played like a champion. No chance of that now, of course, but I can still dream, and managed to achieve my main objective in a career that has been both interesting and completely absorbing.

True to his word – usually a Gaelic one which I never understand! – Niall MacFarlane and I went at the beginning of the week to try his golf buggy as a passenger around some of the golf holes at the Royal Burgess Golf Club. This demonstrated that I could easily and comfortably get in and out of the buggy and putt! Actually, I sank the first putt I tried, at a distance of ten feet and on a slope, which surprised us both and pleased me! I did, however, find gripping the shaft of the putter very difficult, with the tendency of my right hand to 'claw'. This will be something for me to work on if I wish to progress on to chipping, as it will require a better grip. It also was a great thrill to be once more out on golf course again with some hope for the future, even though it would in all likelihood be restricted and I would have to use a buggy to get about.

In the afternoon, Moira accompanied me in what was the longest measured walk so far from our house to the paper shop via the now being demolished Barnton Hotel – fifty minutes, 3,285 steps and 3.18 kilometres, which is almost two miles. Translated into golf holes, this might be about six to eight on an average course without using a buggy. Talking about sport and great achievement, it is notable that Tiger Woods has just won the prestigious American Professional Open Golf Tournament in spite of a painful knee after recent surgery. This was his fourteenth major tournament win, but he still has a few more to get before he can beat the record of my personally greatest sporting hero – Jack Nicklaus, the 'Golden Bear'. Great news from South America: Scotland have managed to win their second test rugby match against Argentina – the first time they have managed to do this in Argentina. Well done! Finally, Allan McNish, a Scot from Dumfries, was one of the drivers who won the 24-hour Le Mans endurance race in a triumph of skill, speed, and endurance.

The tree blossoms such as cherry and laburnum have gone or, in the case of the latter, are certainly on the wane. The main colour in the gardens seems to be provided by roses, poppies and various shrubs, while the birds seem to be a little less visible and vocal. Perhaps this is because of the cold weather or because their young have all fled their nests. We believe that some baby blue tits successfully fledged from the garden nest box during the previous week, and have caught glimpses of them in the oak trees as they called out to be fed.

Flaming June? As I write this it is cold and raining... Let's hope that the second half will be better!

Royal Ascot and Wimbledon Fortnight
(but not forgetting the Highland Show)

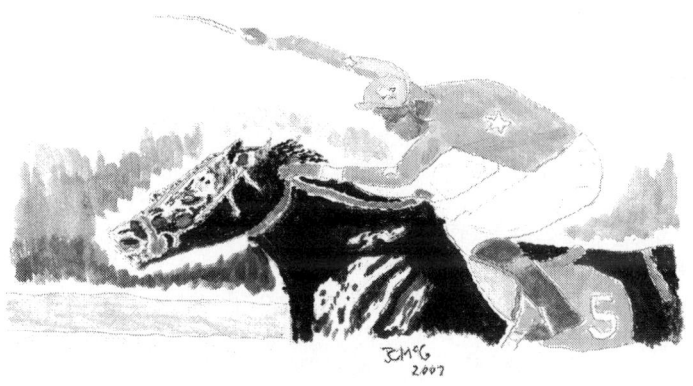

The last few weeks of June are full of events that typify being
'British' and, in the case of the latter, being Scottish. Royal
Ascot, a horse racing event lasting five days, is characterised by
the presence of the Queen, the best horses and jockeys, and
formal dress code, with the ladies dressing up in fine frocks
and fancy hats. Not really my cup of tea, but as seen on
television in small doses quite a colourful and interesting sight.
I watched some of this and enjoyed the opening ceremonies
and was stimulated to go out and walk non-stop the whole way
around our estate, beating the record of the previous day –
3,550 steps in fifty minutes – 3.44 kilometres, which is just
over two miles! Later this week the annual Highland Show
opens at the Ingliston Showground just outside Edinburgh,
and hopefully the weather will be good, as it always proves to
be a very popular attraction for both farming and non-farming
people. I have in the past visited and have had a very interesting
experience but I doubt, given that a lot of walking would be
required to make the most of a visit, if I will go this year.

Fortunately, some of the highlights will be shown on the television. What would I do without it!

What would I do without the newspapers? Probably I could manage, given the almost complete coverage of sport and politics on the many television programmes. I still have difficulty holding and turning the pages of the larger papers but they are still useful for local and Scottish news. They are always a good, though sometimes controversial, source of medical stories and information. At the present time the main medical stories relate to such things as genetic engineering, ways to lose weight and look younger with cosmetic products and surgery, hospital acquired infections such as MRSA and clostridium difficile, vaccination of young school girls against cervical cancer, the high costs and the justification for NHS treatment of patients with terminal conditions, and care of the aged and those with disabilities. Many of the new innovations and treatments are controversial as well as confusing but make interesting reading; no doubt they are seen by the editors to be a good way of maintaining sales!

There are many articles on diet and the benefits or otherwise of different foods I was interested in one such written by David Grotto in the *Daily Mail* on 17 June and extracted from his book, *101 Foods That Could Save Your Life*. Amongst other things, and relevant to me, I read that strawberries were useful in anti-clotting in animals and controlled type 2 diabetes by reducing blood glucose levels after a starchy meal. Potato peel can also reduce blood sugar levels in diabetics, as can asparagus and figs. Eating an egg first thing in the morning may lead to reduced calorie consumption over the rest of the day and thus help to prevent obesity.

The television this week is filled with the continuing games in the finals of the European football championships, but as there are no British teams competing it is less of a spectacle as yet. The most interesting programme so far was one of several that followed the successful three-week series which I enjoyed greatly and have already alluded to – *Springwatch*. These were shown on week nights during the week by each of the main presenters. I particularly enjoyed the hour-long programme by Simon King and the scenes of wild boar in the south of England and the rutting red deer on a Scottish island. His quiet yet informative presentations, coupled with his undoubted enthusiasm, are magical in a totally different way from the approach of the real masters of natural history presentation – David Attenborough and his team. One interesting thing I learned from the programmes was that recordings of the dawn chorus were used in the Alder Hey Children's Hospital to help anxious children relax, and Simon feels 'that the melodious song of the blackbird will remove the forehead wrinkles of anyone who is stressed or worried'. I certainly agree with that sentiment. Incidentally, there is still a dawn chorus to hear, starting at about 3.15 a.m. and made up predominantly of blackbirds, with the first singer often being a song thrush. A strange and almost sinister silence then occurs from about 4 a.m. – probably time for looking for food.

The weekly visit to the gym and the swimming pool went well and, although I am not yet able to be sure, I think my shoulder has become less consistently sore and possibly more mobile. The buoyancy in the pool has definitely helped in my ability to move both my leg and arm with less discomfort.

My walks at the end of this week were conducted in windy conditions so I had to be careful that I did not stumble, but I managed fine, though it was quite challenging. I think that the pedometer showed that I was taking more and shorter steps, as to be expected. Two new walks were done though only one was measured. The first was a walk twice around the nearby Blackhall Park and measured 1,429 steps and about three-quarters of a mile. I did this while Moira took Holly to the adjacent swing park.

The second walk was on the following day – 21 June, the longest day of the year – and fortunately taken in the early afternoon, before the heavy rain later in the evening and the cold temperature made it feel winter had arrived! This walk was around the recently improved Inverleith Park pond, with ducks, mute swans, and moorhens swimming happily in much cleaner water, with an attractive area at one side filled artistically with yellow flowering water irises. According to a notice information board, the park was first opened in 1890 and was to enable people the chance of being able to enjoy fresh air and open countryside. It was of some interest that the recent work done to revive the pond was organised by Nick Benge, who had been involved in setting up and maintaining our tropical fish tank in the sitting room at home.

A bit of excitement came earlier in the day when our son, Alan, telephoned from Bangalore in India to tell us that he would be coming home with Susanna and grandson, Joshua, in about fourteen days' time. This was something to look forward to, especially as it was intended to be a permanent move for a few years. Fortunately, Alan has a flat in Edinburgh, but initially they will be able to stay with us.

An item of news was the 'exciting' information that 'water has been found on Mars' and this was 'a major breakthrough in the search for life in space'. This has just been discovered by NASA's Phoenix probe, which has successfully landed on the planet. The actual capability of the scientists and mathematicians to send a probe to Mars, and successfully land and instruct it, represents the true brilliance of modern mankind. This made me reflect on some of the remaining mysteries, and what I would consider to be the outstanding achievement of man during my own lifetime. With regard to the latter, while the computer, the mobile phone, 'hybrid' cars and fuels, tissue transplantation and microsurgery are great developments, the sending of men to the moon and their safe return to Earth in July 1969 remains for me the greatest of all. As the first man who landed and stood on the moon, Neil Armstrong said, 'That's one small step for man, one giant leap for mankind!' 1969 was also a memorable year for British sport – Tony Jacklin became only the second Briton since Max Faulkner in 1951 to become the British Open Golf Champion, and Ann Jones won the Wimbledon Tennis Singles Championship to become the second British person since World War II to do so. Of even greater importance to me personally, was the fact that I graduated in medicine in June of that year and started my first job in August! What about the mysteries that remain and probably will stay so? I would dearly like to solve these, but part of me says that it would be better to leave them alone and keep them for something to speculate and debate on. I can mention briefly my own thoughts. Here are my ten most keen questions:

1. Where does mankind originate from, and did Man evolve as Darwin suggests from ape-like beings – or did we arrive on Earth from an outside world?

2. Will Man survive on Earth for more than a few generations more, and what are my own distant origins?

3. What happened to cause the demise of the dinosaurs – was it due to severe climate change caused by a large meteorite crashing on Earth, or something else?

4. Do UFOs exist or are they simply optical illusions?

5. Do the Yeti and similar animals like the Loch Ness monster and Bigfoot actually exist, or are they simply fictitious and a production to promote the tourist industry?

6. Why were the pyramids constructed, and what is the significance of their geometry and mathematical constructions?

7. Is the year 2009 predicted to be a year of major World disasters? See point 9 below!

8. How and why were the large standing stone structures in Orkneys, Stonehenge, and other parts of Britain constructed?

9. Does climate change occur as a result of increased carbon dioxide in the atmosphere, or as part of a normal cyclical weather change which coincides with a change in the Earth's polarity, which apparently is due to occur in 2009? This was an interesting theory which I read about several years ago and was based on a retrospective analysis of major disasters in the world over thousands of years and connected by a change in the Earth's polarity.

10. Are we alone in the universe, or are there living creatures elsewhere?

It seems that though I now have lots of time to think about these matters, I am no closer to answering these difficult questions and I have to concentrate on my own particular physical problems! However, with regard to the question of my own origins, I made some progress in my investigations using both conventional professional methods of tracing ancestors and chromosome analysis studies with genetic interpretation. It appeared that on my father's side, most of the older relatives on the male side were either shoemakers or hairdressers, while on my mother's side they were mostly farmers or worked on farms. There was a slight possibility of being related to a Galloway titled family called Herries, who once owned important land and property, and being related thereby to the character in Sir Walter Scott's novel called *Redgauntlet* – said to have been a real person!

The results of the genetic study were performed in Oxford, following sending a buccal smear sample by post. These were extremely interesting! The use of DNA studies has recently become a useful means of investigation in criminology, archaeology, and in the study of population origins and composition. Analysis of my Y chromosome revealed that I am descended from the Celts found predominately in Ireland and Northern and Western Britain and linked to some of the earliest inhabitants who arrived in Britain about 10,000 years ago. As high proportions of similar genetic material in are found in Basques, there may have been seaborne traffic in ancient times between Britain and the Atlantic seaboard of Spain and France. Analysis of on my maternal side using DNA analysis of mitochondria indicated that I am descended from a European woman who originated in the tundra on the eastern edge of the Black Sea. When the Ice Age came there was a migration east and west, spreading all over Europe and even into North America, which suggests that they travelled across Asia and went into the Americas via the then dry Bering land bridge.

Talking about physical problems, Wimbledon fortnight has just started and most, if not all, British hopes rest with the Scot, Andrew Murray, who has had his fair share of injuries. The weather forecast for the tennis is always of interest, and for the first few days at least the sun has been shining in London (and Andy won his first match!). Golf has injury problems as well; Tiger Woods won recently in America, although he required a play-off and he did this with severe discomfort due to left knee ligament problem and a stress fracture in his leg. These injuries, caused by his sport, mean he will not play in the British Open or in the Ryder Cup later this year.

I went to the gym and swimming pool this week and probably made my good arm and leg sore following a try at the vibrator machine, which involved me in getting down on the floor and then getting up again! Hopefully this will get better as it definitely affecting my comfort in walking. I do not think I will be trying this again!

At the recommendation of Betty, we arranged a home visiting physiotherapist to come and assess me. Although I am very happy with the help already given to me by Julie Hooper, this is continuing less often and probably only for a limited time. The new physiotherapist, Emma, came to see me and, after an assessment, arranged for some new exercises and suggested it might be worthwhile buying an extra finger splint, which Jim and Lenny had already got. She showed me a power point presentation on the splint and its use with patients who, before using it, were unable to pick up and release objects. I decided to go ahead and try the apparatus, which apparently is made to order in the USA. Accordingly, Emma carefully made measurements of my finger sizes, wrist, and mid-forearm diameters prior to making an order. She felt as I already had reasonable dexterity in my affected hand I should be able to make good progress.

On the last Saturday of the month, Moira and I travelled through to Glasgow by car for Jean and Graeme Smith's Ruby Wedding Anniversary celebration held at the Cathcart Castle Golf Club. This couple were one of our first new friends when we were first married and lived in the same area. We stayed the night at the Holiday Inn in East Kilbride and had a very enjoyable time. The following day we went to see Jean and Graeme in their house in Newton Mearns, had lunch, and took the opportunity of visiting our first house nearby in the Crookfur estate. We were pleased to see after thirty-two years that it was still standing and in good condition – a bit like I hoped to be eventually! I had a very interesting discussion with Graeme, who has written and hopes to publish a book entitled *The Theatre Royal: Entertaining a Nation* in September 2008. It is the story of Glasgow's famous Theatre Royal and will be produced in full colour, with 280 pages and around 400 illustrations of the people, performances and city it grew up with. To save costs he has planned to publish the book himself – something which I had not myself considered.

The final of the European Football Championship between Spain and Germany also occurred on the Sunday, and this was an intriguing match, won by Spain by 1–0, demonstrating the skill and team tactics required to defeat an inferior and confident opponent. Apparently, this was the first major tournament victory for Spain after forty-four years and laid to rest the label 'non-achievers', which reflected success at club level compared to relative failures at international competitions.

The last day of June was dull in Edinburgh but hot and sunny for Wimbledon, where Andy Murray, the last remaining British singles competitor in the tournament, played a fourth round match and won in a thrilling five-set match. He now plays Rafael Nadal – the second seed and a formidable opponent – in two days' time in the quarter-finals.

Worryingly, my left leg is still sore on walking, and it appears to be related to the calf muscles; hopefully it will get better soon.

The Year is almost Up – I'm Still Here!

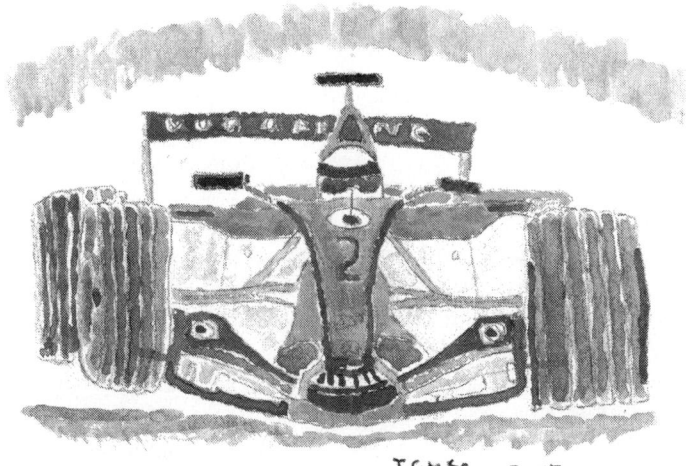

JCMᶜG 2007

On the first of July, Moira and I went to St John's Hospital in West Lothian to see Linda, my last secretary, and any of the other staff who were present in the regional Plastic Surgery Unit. This was to be the first time I had visited since my stroke and also since retiring from the NHS in April 2006. Naturally, I viewed the visit with mixed emotions, but I needn't have worried as I was made very welcome and we were given coffee and biscuits. I also enjoyed meeting other secretaries, Fay and Valerie, as well as charge nurses, Chris from ward 20 – the Burn Unit – and Val from ward 18. Various others spoke to me, including ward orderlies, Patrick Armstrong, one of the newest plastic surgery Consultants, and one of the members of the photographic team who in the past has been of great help to me in my presentations and publications. The general view was that I looked well and had lost some weight! The journey there and back by car reminded me of the many journeys I used to make, and although the scenery is mostly in the countryside, it is not one that I miss now, particularly as these trips were often done in very busy traffic conditions when I rarely had time to enjoy the scenery. At this time I noticed the dog rose shrubs with their pink flowers at the sides of the roads, together with the profusion of grasses, buttercups, clover flowers, hemlocks, yellow ragwort, pink rose bay willowherb, and the occasional foxgloves and red poppies in the verges.

My right arm and leg remained sore and my walking seemed definitely affected. As I was slightly concerned in case I had developed a deep vein thrombosis, and Moira was also worried, we decided to visit the GP for advice. We saw Dr Jolliffe and he considered that I had muscle strains and there were no signs to suggest deep vein thrombosis – much to my relief! He advised that I reduce my activities for a few days and accordingly, I cancelled my next gym visit and planned to stop trying to beat time and distance records in my various walks – at least for a week or so! I planned to concentrate on those exercises that could be done in the house and to try to wear the SaeboStretch splint for longer periods of time. It does show me how important it is to preserve the function of the unaffected limbs for anyone who has a stroke and how important it is to avoid falling and injuring or even sustaining a fracture. Hence the great concern in hospital if any patient falls and the checks before going home made by the occupational therapy team of the patient's home to see potential problems and arrange for handrails or any other modifications that might be required.

Yes, I am still here, unlike our tennis hero! Andy Murray was soundly defeated in three sets by the muscular, very fit, and brilliant Nadal, who must be one of the favourites to win this year's Wimbledon Singles Title. Still, in reaching the quarter-finals, Andy has shown he has the potential of one day achieving greatness and giving the British public something to be proud of. These indeed are hard times, what with a high inflation rate, falling house values, difficulties for the first time buyers with mortgages, as well as rising food, gas/electrical and petrol/diesel costs. Sport has the great capacity of inspiring and elevating the spirit of the spectator as well as the participants. For me and my recovery, I can certainly vouch for the former and for the latter in a much more modified capacity!

Since I was purposely not trying for a few days to go for long walks, I took the opportunity of sitting in our back garden and noticed during the sunny afternoon much less bird activity at our bird feeders and less birdsong. No longer were there the sounds of robins, chaffinches, wrens and greenfinches, or even hedge sparrows.

Visits to the feeders were infrequent and were usually coal or blue tits. The main and very melodious songsters were the blackbirds, who seemed to start up and increase in numbers as they appeared to answer and compete with each other. The other interesting thing that I noticed was a grey squirrel sitting on the trunk of an oak tree, uttering curious rasping sounds and flicking its tail. I am not sure what the significance of this is. As before there was no evidence of honeybees but plenty of bumblebees. I also saw no butterflies, but it is possible that at present our garden has not yet got flowers that would attract them. In the front garden, which I look out on each day, I have enjoyed watching a robin on the lawn and seeing it frequently using a perch on the head of a small 'Peter Pan' statue in our front border. This has given me an idea for a possible Christmas card painting in due course. My collection of cacti are or have been flowering and as usual there has been several stunning and beautiful blooms; given their jaggy and intimidating appearance, this remains a very pleasing attribute particularly as they require surprisingly little care throughout the year. During the one short walk I took outside, I smelled a very pleasant odour which emanated from a large bush of flowering honeysuckle growing in a nearby garden – something that was not a feature of my cacti flowers.

5 July is the actual sixtieth anniversary of the start of the NHS, and in the evening on BBC 2 there was a very interesting documentary on its origins and the considerable debate at the time between the doctors and the Conservative opponents, including Sir Winston Churchill, and Bevan. The doctors, who were largely opposed, were brought into line by the promise of being able to keep, if wished, the right to private practice. Initially,

the change to free treatment resulted in a huge increase in the numbers requesting medication and treatment costs, which was something which threatened to swamp the new arrangement; interestingly, this is exactly what has proved to be a significant issue today. The good thing about the new system was that medical treatments were now freely available to the poorer families, the elderly, and children. Diseases like measles, tuberculosis, diphtheria, and poliomyelitis could now be treated and immunisation programmes started.

It was a dull and wet day in Edinburgh – quite a contrast with the glorious sunshine in London, where Venus Williams defeated her sister Serena in the Ladies' Singles Final. Both won the Ladies' Doubles Final, and a fourteen-year-old girl, Laura Robson, won the Junior Singles Title. Though born in Australia, she has apparently adopted British citizenship, so she has created great excitement in Britain as a future senior champion. Time will tell whether she will have the luck and personality to make 'the big time'. The major sporting interests tomorrow will be the Final of the Men's Singles between the five times in a row winner, Roger Federer, and the clay court maestro, Rafael Nadal. Of additional interest will be the British Grand Prix Formula 1 racing car championship, in which Lewis Hamilton, a British hopeful, will participate. The winner of the tennis was Nadal, after a five-set epic, while Lewis Hamilton won the British Grand Prix.

The most exciting thing for me and Moira on the evening of this day – 6 July – is the arrival of Alan, Susanna, and grandson Joshua John McGregor from India at Edinburgh Airport. It is planned that initially they will stay with us, and in the long term they aim to stay in the UK for several years. They arrived to be met by Moira, and a 'dreich' wet Scottish welcome! Quite a contrast to Bangalore from whence they had come.

This day was also the twentieth anniversary of the Piper Alpha oil rig fire and disaster just off Aberdeen, in which over 160 persons died. Having been involved in the care of burns, and having campaigned to prevent the closure of the regional Burn Unit in Bangour and St John's Hospital, West Lothian, I can well appreciate what happened and the bravery of those involved. I hope we will never face another such problem in the future, though I am pleased that in my working career I helped to prevent the Unit's closure. I also published my concerns that Scotland may not be fully prepared for a major disaster in which burn casualties were a major concern, and how this could be helped. (*Journal of the Royal College of Surgeons of Edinburgh and Ireland*, 2004)

During the first week of this month I had my first driving lesson as part of the plan to be able to drive again. This was a daunting prospect, even though I had had a successful testing at Astley Ainslie a few months ago. Firstly, there would be a new instructor, a new car, and – horror of horrors – I would be unleashed to the outside public roads after an absence of twelve months! The Vauxhall car came to collect me at home and was accompanied by a very helpful and experienced lady instructor, Ann, who specialised in instructing people like me. The car could be fitted with various devices to aid the driver, and in my case a steering wheel control for my left hand was added to the steering wheel, and this also had wiper, horn, indicators, and light controls that could be operated by my left thumb. It was confirmed that I could use my left foot on the brake pedal and my right foot with the ankle support on the accelerator pedal. A successful two-hour lesson went well, and a further lesson to increase my experience was booked for a week ahead. It was certainly a great morale-booster to be able to drive again – albeit under instruction.

There is no doubt I have torn some muscle in my good leg and this has been making walking more painful and also tricky while coming down stairs. There has been some improvement over about a week, and Moira has noticed some bruising which has become more noticeable to me on the inner aspect of my lower leg on 10 July. I have been able to wear my hand splint each day for up to six hours and do some of the shoulder exercises, but have not been this week to the gym or swimming pool; this has possibly helped my recovery, in that I rested the affected leg, but it would have been difficult because of our relatives staying with us while they try to sort out their affairs with our help. There has also been the additional interest and some stress in the household as a new fireplace has just been installed in our sitting room, and various furniture shifts has had to be done. No doubt it will be an attractive addition to our house, and it is something that Moira has wanted for a long time – she certainly has deserved it!

Alan, Susanna, and Joshua stayed with us for six days and left to go to their own flat in town. We enjoyed their stay and of course seeing young Joshua taking his first steps. On the day they left we took Callum to a local play park and then to the Gyle Shopping Centre for the 'promised' ice cream, which I admit I also enjoyed! This day, as it happens, was exactly one week before the anniversary date of my stroke one year ago, and to prove my fitness was recovering well after the problem with my left leg, I was able to walk the full circuit of over one mile around our area without any problem. It was quite noticeable that there were fewer birds singing – the occasional wren, crow, and squadrons of jackdaws flying about. I wondered why there were so many jackdaws and where their colonies were to be found, as to the best of my knowledge they usually nest in old ruined buildings – none of which are to be found nearby.

During the week that Alan stayed I read one of two books he had given me to read, entitled *Stupid White Men* by Michael Moore. This is a strange non-fictional book described as 'savagely hilarious', and is only available uncensored because of public pressure which forced publication in the face of what seemed to be serious criticism of George Bush, the background voting system, the policies with regard to the environment, education, libraries, the penal system, and the treatment of women and the black population. I must admit that it was quite an astonishing and slightly funny book which did not hold back in its views. Certainly quite thought provoking, but not a book to be read by the faint-hearted! The second book, which I started to read after this and planned to complete before the end of my own account, was *Freakonomics* by Levitt and Dubner. It is an equally thought-provoking book, in which a rogue economist explores the 'hidden side of everything' and certainly introduced some interesting ideas on a number of topical issues in life. This was certainly a riveting read for someone like me and, although it might be associated with the title of this book, my experience was completely different!

The last few days before my one-year anniversary of my stroke involved a visit to see Julie at McLeod Street where I was told that, according to previous measurements, I had significantly improved my right shoulder mobility and should now try to improve on hand functions. I also had a second driving lesson and moved out onto more busy roads without obvious problems and, of more significance, had my first fall since my discharge from hospital. It was outside in our garden while trying to come down some steps – probably due to my still sore left calf, and poor or careless use of my walking stick. I was certain that I neither felt dizzy nor fainted. Fortunately, I received only minor knee and elbow abrasions, some vague discomfort on my right chest, and a 'rollicking' from a very concerned Moira. Indeed, this was a salutary and extremely valuable lesson to me, but illustrated what problems could still occur for the unwary.

Towards the end of this last week, the British Open golf tournament begins at Royal Birkdale and I look forward to the usually excellent TV coverage. At the weekend Moira and I will be back in Inverurie to see Moira's mother and will probably 'celebrate' the anniversary on that day – 19 July!

The trip up to Inverurie went well, even though the journey up was made in extremely gusty and wet conditions. It was also unseasonably cold. Again, we stayed overnight in the Strathburn Hotel, and Moira was able to do various things to help her mother. The return journey was in much sunnier conditions and again I enjoyed looking at the countryside and roadside plants. In particular I noticed the lack of the golden colour provided by the broom which had now ceased to flower but the white banks of ox-eye daisies, the patches of creamy white meadowsweets, and the pink rosebay willowherb provided interesting as well as colourful replacements.

The climax to the weekend, and to my own 'year', was the last day of the British Open Golf Championship held near Liverpool and won by Padraig Harrington – he had also won last year! The television presentation was as usual well done and, for someone like me unable to walk long distances, it really offers an ideal way of seeing most players and the drama that always occurs.

One Year On: What are my Lessons and Messages?

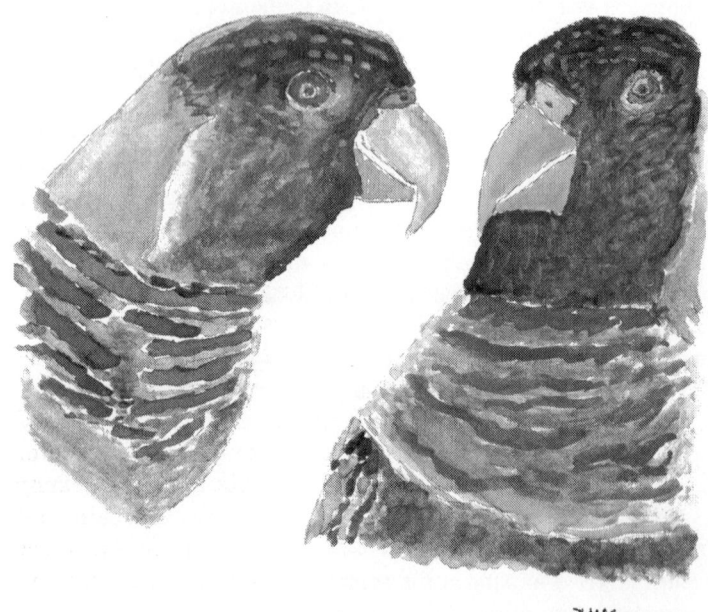

A pair of parakeets

It seems unbelievable to think back one year ago and reflect on the progress made in that time! I still feel that there are still some things that can be improved, especially with regard to function of my right hand and shoulder. These, I appreciate, can be slower than any recovery in the affected leg in the stroke person, and may only achieve 'normality' in about 25% of cases – but I am determined to try to achieve this! Hopefully, the exercises and splints organised by Julie and Emma will help me to work on these aspects. I have been fortunate in having had excellent initial care in the hospitals, first class outpatient and home care, but perhaps more than anything, a wonderful carer – Moira. The devotion and loyal commitment of the carer is undoubtedly a key to my success and happiness, and was also seen with the wives of Lenny and Jim, with whom we have become soulmates and mutual advisors on various problems. The great thing is to try and achieve a balance between the natural concern of the helpers and the desire of the patient to be allowed to be more adventurous and independent.

In spite of this I still feel frustrated that I am not as mobile and helpful to Moira as I used to be, but I am lucky that I have no mental or language problems with my type of stroke, and also I have had no facial weakness; clearly these are situations which can make the care and recovery from a stroke much more of a problem for the sufferer as well as the carers. I also acknowledge that being relatively well off and medically knowledgeable has been extremely helpful under difficult circumstances, and the latter has given me a unique insight into strokes.

There is no doubt in my mind that, apart from a belief that I could eventually get better, even if there was an element of uncertainty about the degree of improvement, it was something that motivated me to keep on trying. By reading, watching TV programmes, listening to music, writing this book and other articles, an increased interest in natural history, re-learning to walk and drive, and finding that I could draw and paint with my unaffected non-dominant hand, I was able to fill in my time as well as possibly aid my recovery. I felt my life was still worthwhile!

The ability to be able to draw and paint, which before the stroke I had no particular skill or desire to do, was a real surprise to me, and gave me much pleasure as well as the suggesting the title for this book. Whether I had developed a degree of being ambidextrous as a result of my surgical background or the stroke itself caused some releasing effect on my unaffected right brain, this for me seems to be the most surprising result of all. One of the most pleasant and stimulating things apart from the above has been the fun and presence of my grandchildren, Callum, Holly, and Joshua, whose antics and energy have established a purpose and continuity of family life which I have valued greatly. I look forward to the birth of a fourth grandchild next month – this will be Trudy's third child!

As I was about to retire from private surgical practice and had already left the NHS, being unable to return to my work because of my stroke affected me to a lesser extent than it might have done. I had to withdraw from some of my other medical duties, including various committees and examining commitments, many of which I enjoyed. There was some hope that I might some day be able to return to a few of these and I have been encouraged by an approach from the Edinburgh College of Surgeons representative, Mr Pradip Datta, with regard to undertaking some examining duties in the nearby Western General Hospital in the autumn.

I have also been encouraged in that I have been asked again to be a reviewer for articles submitted to the *Journal of Plastic and Aesthetic Surgery* and have one, possibly two, articles accepted for publication in the same prestigious journal. One of these was written and submitted while I was recovering in hospital using my portable personal computer. This was a most valuable addition to the things that helped me pass the time, feel in some control of my life, and of course enabled me to keep a record of events as a diary, which formed the basis of material for a book. There was no problem in using one hand, while the odd occasions when two were required were not usually beyond me or a sympathetic relative.

Another matter that I have become adjusted to with some initial unhappiness has been the change in diet – no or low salt intake, no sugar, and low fat – but here I have managed to accommodate. It means an end to crisps, lashings of butter, eggs, and frequent high sugar content soft drinks. Moira makes sure that I stick to the rules!

I used to think that strokes were a sign of and unique preserve of the old, but since being afflicted and considering myself as relatively young and fit beforehand, I have seen and met several people younger than myself who have had a stroke. In fact about thirty per cent of strokes occur in persons aged less than sixty to sixty-five years of age, and in some cases in very young people or even children. The predisposing factors associated include high blood pressure, diabetes, several drugs, and congenital and hereditary history. With an ageing population, the increased incidence of these as well as atherosclerosis makes the incidence of strokes more common. Fortunately, this has been recognised and much research into the causes as well as the aftercare is now in progress in the UK.

Could I have predicted or reduced the chances of a stroke in my case? Firstly, there was nothing in my family history which suggested I was at risk including diabetes, and both my parents lived until the age of ninety years. Both did, however, suffer from ischaemic heart disease and this contributed to their ill health and eventual death. I was a non-smoker, and although both my parents did smoke they managed to stop in their latter years. Passively, as a child, I probably was subjected to a fair amount of cigarette smoke in the house.

In the last few years before my stroke, I had two or three episodes of nosebleeds, which could have been a symptom of high blood pressure, but no headaches. I did seem to be drinking more water during my clinics and during breaks in my operating sessions, but thought this was due to the hot environment in the hospitals. Increased and urgent toilet visits were I thought simply a normal ageing process! Because I had never been ill and never been off work during all the time I worked in the NHS and for the extra year I worked in private practice, I was lulled into a false feeling that I was completely healthy as well as indestructible, even though at times I felt more tired than usual. I put this down to 'getting older'.

Surprisingly, even though I was a doctor, I failed to take account of several curious episodes of dizziness, double vision, and increased sweating attacks which preceded my stroke in the months beforehand. I now know these were what are termed 'transient ischaemic episodes' or TIEs. Whether, had I gone earlier to seek medical advice, I would have changed the course of my illness or not remains for ever unknown, but my advice to others would be that they should.

Strokes will continue to happen unexpectedly, even when

predisposing factors are known. I hope my personal account will be a help to carers and patients alike in coping with what is truly a life-changing experience.

Bibliography

Bryson, Bill, *Down Under*, MacMillan, London, 2001

——, *Shakespeare*, HarperPress, London, 2007

Bruce, George, *Through the Letterbox: Haikus*, Renaissance Press, 2001

'Chest, Heart, and Stroke', Fact sheets, 2006, 65 North Castle Street, Edinburgh EH2 3LT, www.chss.org.uk

Grotto, David, *101 Foods That Could Save Your Life*, Bantam, 2008

Harris, Rolf, *Rolf on Art*, BBC Worldwide Ltd, 2002

Levitt, Steven D, and Dubner, Stephen J, *Freakonomics*, Harper-Collins, New York, New York 10022, 2006

McCann, Nick, *Balmoral: Guide to the Castle and Estate*, Heritage House Group Ltd, Derby, 2007

McCrum, Robert, *My Year Off*, Picador/MacMillan, London, 1998

McGregor, John C, 'Turn to the left', *Surgeons' News*, Volume 7, pp.57–8, April 2008

——, 'Major Burn Disasters – Lessons to be learned from previous incidents and a need for a National Plan. Matter for debate', *Journal of the Royal College of Surgeons of Edinburgh and Ireland*, vols. 2–5, pp.249–250, 2004

Moore, Michael, *Stupid White Men*, Penguin Books Ltd, London, 1994

O'Hare, Mick, *Why Don't Penguins' Feet Freeze?* Profile Books Ltd, London, 2006

Rodgers, Helen, and Thomson, Richard, Editorial, 'Functional status and long term outcome of stroke', *British Medical Journal*, Volume 336, 16 February 2008

Rose, Gareth, 'Now stroke victims get a Wii bit of extra help', *Evening News*, 15 May 2008

Smith, Elisabeth, *Instant Spanish*, Hodder Education, London, 2006

Smith, Graeme, *The Theatre Royal: Entertaining a Nation*, Glasgow Publications, Glasgow, 2008

Stephen, Martin, *Diary of a Stroke*, Psychology News Press, 2008

Stewart, Paul D, *Galapagos: The Islands that Changed the World*, BBC Books, 2006

Taylor, Kenny, *Scotland's Nature and Wildlife*, Lomond Books, Edinburgh, 2002

Trees and Shrubs of Britain, The Reader's Digest Association Ltd, London, 1981

Turner, Barry, *The Writers' Handbook 2008*, Macmillan Ltd, 2007

Vallely, Joanna, 'Rising temperatures put the heat on for Capital's wild life', *Evening News*, 20 February 2008

White, Michael, *Leonardo: The First Scientist*, Abacus, London, 2000

Wildlife of Britain, Midsummer Group Ltd, London, 2007

Printed in Great Britain
by Amazon.co.uk, Ltd.,
Marston Gate.